Beyond LC-MS: The Next Frontier in Clinical Mass Spectrometry

Editor

SANKHA S. BASU

CLINICS IN LABORATORY MEDICINE

www.labmed.theclinics.com

Editor-in-Chief
MILENKO JOVAN TANASIJEVIC

June 2021 • Volume 41 • Number 2

ELSEVIER

1600 John F. Kennedy Boulevard • Suite 1800 • Philadelphia, Pennsylvania, 19103-2899

http://www.theclinics.com

CLINICS IN LABORATORY MEDICINE Volume 41, Number 2
June 2021 ISSN 0272-2712, ISBN-13: 978-0-323-81329-7

Editor: Katerina Heidhausen
Developmental Editor: Ann Gielou M. Posedio

Reprints. For copies of 100 or more, of articles in this publication, please contact the Commercial Reprints Department, Elsevier Inc., 360 Park Avenue South, New York, New York 10010-1710. Tel. 212-633-3874, Fax: 212-633-3820, E-mail: reprints@elsevier.com.

Clinics in Laboratory Medicine (ISSN 0272-2712) is published quarterly by Elsevier Inc., 360 Park Avenue South, New York, NY 10010-1710. Months of issue are March, June, September, and December. Business and Editorial offices: 1600 John F. Kennedy Blvd., Suite 1800, Philadelphia, PA 19103-2899. Periodicals postage paid at NewYork, NY and additional mailing offices. Subscription prices are $283.00 per year (US individuals), $731.00 per year (US institutions), $100.00 per year (US students), $363.00 per year (Canadian individuals), $768.00 per year (Canadian institutions), $100.00 per year (Canadian students), $404.00 per year (international individuals), $768.00 per year (international institutions), $185.00 (international students). Foreign air speed delivery is included in all Clinics subscription prices. All prices are subject to change without notice. POSTMASTER: Send address changes to *Clinics in Laboratory Medicine*, Elsevier Health Sciences Division, Subscription Customer Service, 3251 Riverport Lane, Maryland Heights, MO 63043. **Customer Service: 1-800-654-2452 (US). From outside of the US and Canada, call 1-314-447-8871. Fax: 1-314-447-8029. E-mail: journalscustomerservice-usa@elsevier.com (for print support) or journalsonlinesupport-usa@elsevier.com (for online support).**

Clinics in Laboratory Medicine is covered in *EMBASE/Exerpta Medica, MEDLINE/PubMed (Index Medicus), Cinahl, Current Contents/Clinical Medicine, BIOSIS and ISI/BIOMED.*

Contributors

EDITOR-IN-CHIEF

MILENKO JOVAN TANASIJEVIC, MD, MBA
Vice Chair for Clinical Pathology and Quality, Department of Pathology, Director of Clinical Laboratories, Brigham and Women's Hospital, Dana-Farber Cancer Institute, Associate Professor of Pathology, Harvard Medical School, Boston, Massachusetts, USA

EDITOR

SANKHA S. BASU, MD, PhD
Assistant Director of Clinical Chemistry and Mass Spectrometry, Department of Pathology, Brigham and Women's Hospital, Instructor of Pathology, Harvard Medical School, Boston, Massachusetts

AUTHORS

NATHALIE Y.R. AGAR, PhD
Associate Professor of Neurosurgery and Associate Professor of Radiology, Harvard Medical School, Daniel E. Ponton Distinguished Chair in Neurosurgery, Brigham and Women's Hospital, Boston, Massachusetts, USA

YAZAN AL-JABAWI, MBBS
Division of Infectious Diseases, Brigham and Women's Hospital, Harvard Medical School, Boston, Massachusetts, USA

OBADAH ALOUM, MBBS
Division of Infectious Diseases, Brigham and Women's Hospital, Harvard Medical School, Boston, Massachusetts, USA

PEGGI M. ANGEL, PhD
Assistant Professor, Department of Cell and Molecular Pharmacology, Medical University of South Carolina, Charleston, South Carolina, USA

SANKHA S. BASU, MD, PhD
Assistant Director of Clinical Chemistry and Mass Spectrometry, Department of Pathology, Brigham and Women's Hospital, Instructor of Pathology, Harvard Medical School, Boston, Massachusetts, USA

GREGORY K. BEHBEHANI, MD, PhD
Division of Hematology, Department of Internal Medicine, The Ohio State University Wexner Medical Center, Comprehensive Cancer Center, Columbus, Ohio, USA

ALYSON P. BLACK, BS
Graduate Student, Department of Cell and Molecular Pharmacology, Medical University of South Carolina, Charleston, South Carolina, USA

CALVIN R.K. BLASCHKE, BS
Graduate Student, Department of Cell and Molecular Pharmacology, Medical University of South Carolina, Charleston, South Carolina, USA

CHRISTINE BOLLWEIN, MD
Institute of Pathology, Technical University of Munich, Munich, Germany

CHRISTOPHER R. COX, PhD
Senior Scientist, Cobio Diagnostics, Golden, Colorado, USA

SURENDRA DASARI, PhD
Associate Professor of Biomedical Informatics, Department of Health Sciences Research, Mayo Clinic, Rochester, Minnesota, USA

RAYMOND D. DEVINE, PhD
Division of Hematology, Department of Internal Medicine, The Ohio State University Wexner Medical Center, Comprehensive Cancer Center, Columbus, Ohio, USA

RICHARD R. DRAKE, PhD
Professor, Department of Cell and Molecular Pharmacology, Medical University of South Carolina, Charleston, South Carolina, USA

CHIRANJIT GHOSH, PhD
Division of Infectious Diseases, Brigham and Women's Hospital, Harvard Medical School, Boston, Massachusetts, USA

REBECCA M. HARRIS, MD
Director, Infectious Disease Diagnostics Laboratory, Children's Hospital of Philadelphia, Philadelphia, Pennsylvania, USA

NOUR ISMAIL, MD
Division of Infectious Diseases, Brigham and Women's Hospital, Harvard Medical School, Boston, Massachusetts, USA

LAUREN KATZ, MSc
Techna Institute for the Advancement of Technology for Health, University Health Network, Department of Medical Biophysics, University of Toronto, Toronto, Ontario, Canada

SOPHIA KOO, MD
Division of Infectious Diseases, Brigham and Women's Hospital, Harvard Medical School, Dana-Farber Cancer Institute, Boston, Massachusetts, USA

SEENA KOSHY, PhD
Division of Infectious Diseases, Brigham and Women's Hospital, Harvard Medical School, Boston, Massachusetts, USA

ANNA F. LAU, PhD, D(ABMM)
Chief, Sterility Testing Service, Department of Laboratory Medicine, Clinical Center, National Institutes of Health, Bethesda, Maryland, USA

ARMANDO LEON, MD
Division of Infectious Diseases, Brigham and Women's Hospital, Harvard Medical School, Boston, Massachusetts, USA

JULIANA PEREIRA LOPES GONÇALVES, PhD
Institute of Pathology, Technical University of Munich, Munich, Germany

COLIN T. McDOWELL, BS
Graduate Student, Department of Cell and Molecular Pharmacology, Medical University of South Carolina, Charleston, South Carolina, USA

ANAND S. MEHTA, DPhil
Professor, Department of Cell and Molecular Pharmacology, Medical University of South Carolina, Charleston, South Carolina, USA

DAVID L. MURRAY, MD, PhD
Consultant, Assistant Professor of Laboratory Medicine and Pathology, Department of Laboratory Medicine and Pathology, Mayo Clinic, Rochester, Minnesota, USA

KRISTINA SCHWAMBORN, MD, PhD
Institute of Pathology, Technical University of Munich, Munich, Germany

ALESSANDRA TATA, PhD
Laboratorio di Chimica Sperimentale, Istituto Zooprofilattico delle Venezie, Viale Fiume, Vicenza, Italy

WILKO WEICHERT, MD
Institute of Pathology, Technical University of Munich, Munich, Germany

ZOE FREEMAN WEISS, MD
Division of Infectious Diseases, Brigham and Women's Hospital, Harvard Medical School, Massachusetts General Hospital, Division of Infectious Diseases, Boston, Massachusetts, USA

MICHAEL WOOLMAN, BSc
Techna Institute for the Advancement of Technology for Health, University Health Network, Department of Medical Biophysics, University of Toronto, Toronto, Ontario, Canada

ARASH ZARRINE-AFSAR, PhD
Techna Institute for the Advancement of Technology for Health, University Health Network; Departments of Medical Biophysics and Surgery, University of Toronto; Keenan Research Center for Biomedical Science & the Li Ka Shing Knowledge Institute, St. Michael's Hospital, Toronto, Ontario, Canada

Contents

> Mass spectrometry imaging (MSI) combines the excellence in molecular characterization of mass spectrometry with microscopic imaging capabilities of hematoxylin- and eosin-stained samples, enabling the precise location of several analytes in the tissue. Especially in the field of pathology, MSI may have an impactful role in tumor diagnosis, biomarker identification, prognostic prediction, and characterization of tumor margins during tumor resection procedures. This article discusses the recent developments in the field that are paving the way for this technology to become accepted as an analytical tool in the clinical setting, its current limitations, and future directions.

> Various analytical methods can be applied to concentrate, separate, and examine trace volatile organic metabolites in the breath, with the potential for noninvasive, rapid, real-time identification of various disease processes, including an array of microbial infections. Although biomarker discovery and validation in microbial infections can be technically challenging, it is an approach that has shown great promise, especially for infections that are particularly difficult to identify with standard culture and molecular amplification-based approaches. This article discusses the current state of breath analysis for the diagnosis of infectious diseases.

> The diagnosis of myeloma and other plasma cell disorders has traditionally been done with the aid of electrophoretic methods, whereas amyloidosis has been characterized by immunohistochemistry. Mass spectrometry has recently been established as an alternative to these traditional methods and has been proved to bring added benefit for patient care. These newer mass spectrometry–based methods highlight some of the key advantages of modern proteomic methods and how they can be applied to the routine care of patients.

Rapid characterization of tissue disorder using ambient mass spectrometry (MS) techniques, requiring little to no preanalytical preparations of sampled tissues, has been shown using a variety of ion sources and with many disease classes. A brief overview of ambient MS in clinical applications, the state of the art in regulatory affairs, and recommendations to facilitate adoption for use at the bedside are presented. Unique challenges in the validation of untargeted MS methods and additional safety and compliance requirements for deployment within a clinical setting are further discussed. Development of a harmonized validation strategy for ambient MS methods is emphasized.

N-glycan imaging mass spectrometry (IMS) can rapidly and reproducibly identify changes in disease-associated N-linked glycosylation that are linked with histopathology features in standard formalin-fixed paraffin-embedded tissue samples. It can detect multiple N-glycans simultaneously and has been used to identify specific N-glycans and carbohydrate structural motifs as possible cancer biomarkers. Recent advancements in instrumentation and sample preparation are also discussed. The tissue N-glycan IMS workflow has been adapted to new glass slide–based assays for effective and rapid analysis of clinical biofluids, cultured cells, and immunoarray-captured glycoproteins for detection of changes in glycosylation associated with disease.

Many studies have shown successful performance of matrix-assisted laser desorption ionization time-of-flight mass spectrometry for rapid yeast and mold identification, yet few laboratories have chosen to apply this technology into their routine clinical mycology workflow. This review provides an overview of the current status of matrix-assisted laser desorption ionization time-of-flight mass spectrometry for fungal identification, including key findings in the literature, processing and database considerations, updates in technology, and exciting future prospects. Significant advances toward standardization have taken place recently; thus, accurate species-level identification of yeasts and molds should be highly attainable, achievable, and practical in most clinical laboratories.

Over the past decade, matrix-assisted laser desorption/ionization–time-of-flight mass spectrometry has revolutionized the practice of clinical microbiology and infectious disease diagnostics. Rapid advancement has occurred through the development and implementation of mass spectrometric protein profiling technologies that are widely available. Ease of sample preparation, rapid turnaround times, and high throughput accuracy have accelerated acceptance within the clinical laboratory. New mass spectrometric technologies centered on multiple microbial diagnostic markers are in development. Such new applications, reviewed in this article and on the near horizon, stand to greatly enhance the capabilities and utility for improved mass spectrometric microbial identification and patient care.

Mass cytometry (MC), imaging mass cytometry (IMC), and multiplexed ion beam imaging (MIBI) represent a new generation of tools to understand increasingly complex systems. Although these technologies differ in their intended applications, with MC being most similar to flow cytometry, and IMC/MIBI being similar to immunohistochemistry, they all share a time of flight mass spectrometry (TOF MS) platform. These TOF MS platforms use metal conjugated antibodies as opposed to fluorophores, increasing the measurable parameters up to approximately 50 with a theoretic limit approximately 100 parameters. These tools are being adapted to understand highly complex systems in basic and clinical research.

Matrix-assisted laser desorption/ionization (MALDI) mass spectrometry imaging (MSI) is an emerging analytical technique that promises to change tissue-based diagnostics. This article provides a brief introduction to MALDI MSI as well as clinical diagnostic workflows and opportunities to apply this powerful approach. It describes various MALDI MSI applications, from more clinically mature applications such as cancer to emerging applications such as infectious diseases and drug distribution. In addition, it discusses the analytical parameters that need to be considered when bringing these approaches to different diagnostic problems and settings.

Beyond LC-MS: The Next Frontier in Clinical Mass Spectrometry

CLINICS IN LABORATORY MEDICINE

SERIES OF RELATED INTEREST

Surgical Pathology Clinics
Available at: https://www.surgpath.theclinics.com/

THE CLINICS ARE NOW AVAILABLE ONLINE!
Access your subscription at:
www.theclinics.com

Preface

Beyond LC-MS: The Next Frontier in Clinical Mass Spectrometry

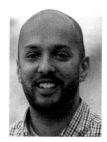

Sankha S. Basu, MD, PhD
Editor

Clinical implementation of mass spectrometry (MS) has been relatively slow compared with nucleic acid and antibody-based methods. Although MS was first described in the early 1900s, it was not applied clinically until the 1970s with gas chromatography, and even then, in a limited capacity. MS saw wider deployment in the 1990s when soft-ionization techniques, such as electrospray ionization, brought together liquid chromatography (LC) and tandem mass spectrometry (MS/MS). The capacity of LC-MS/MS to measure multiple drugs and metabolites quickly and accurately in complex biological matrices solved several diagnostic challenges. Although clinical applications of LC-MS/MS have continued to expand in the ensuing decades, the resources and technical expertise needed to acquire, operate, and maintain these instruments, and laboratory-developed tests have mostly limited it to larger hospital and reference laboratories.

Compared with clinical chemistry, MS utilization in clinical microbiology has seen a steeper rise with the introduction of MALDI-TOF MS for microbial identification. Its broad applicability to routine clinical microbiology workflows, combined with low reagent costs, ease of use, and Food and Drug Administration–approved platforms, has made it easier to adopt in the clinical laboratory. As a result, its uptake has been swift and remarkable, despite only being introduced clinically in the past decade.

In this issue of *Clinics in Laboratory Medicine*, the authors provide an update on some of the exciting progress made using newer MS approaches not only in clinical chemistry and microbiology but also in hematology, immunology, and surgical pathology. It has been a wonderful opportunity to serve as the Guest Editor of this issue and learn more about these developments from leaders in the field. I am also very grateful for their dedication and ability to provide these perspectives during this very challenging pandemic.

On a personal note, much as the field of clinical diagnostics "discovered" MS, many of us who work in clinical MS have our own personal story of "discovering" MS. My

Clin Lab Med 41 (2021) xi–xii
https://doi.org/10.1016/j.cll.2021.03.010
0272-2712/21/© 2021 Published by Elsevier Inc.

journey started in graduate school, when I rotated through a laboratory that happened to have a mass spectrometer. Although my background was in molecular biology, the PI of the laboratory asked if I might be interested working on a lipidomics project using MS. I thought, "Why not? I'll learn something new." In fact, I was so unfamiliar with MS that I reviewed my organic chemistry textbook for a refresher.

I still remember my first day on the instrument, mesmerized by the mass spectra lighting up the screen, as millions of ions whizzed by every millisecond. I was so impressed with the power of the technology that I decided to not only switch the focus of my thesis to MS but also dedicate my professional life to harnessing its potential. My interest only grew deeper during my clinical pathology residency, where I learned how to develop these methods into clinical-grade assays. As a medical microbiology fellow, I was lucky enough to witness the introduction of MALDI-TOF and watch it transform our clinical microbiology workflows seemingly overnight. Finally, as a postdoctoral fellow in Dr Nathalie Agar's laboratory, I was able to experience firsthand the visualization of otherwise invisible metabolism in tissues using mass spectrometry imaging, and the speed afforded by ambient MS opening previously untapped areas such as the operating room.

I have been truly amazed by the clinical potential of MS at every step of my journey, and I hope readers of this issue may find the same inspiration and continue to build bridges between the diagnostics and MS communities.

Sankha S. Basu, MD, PhD
Department of Pathology
Brigham and Women's Hospital
Cotran Building, Room AL.376A
75 Francis St.
Boston, MA 02115, USA

E-mail address:
sbasu@bwh.harvard.edu

Implementation of Mass Spectrometry Imaging in Pathology: Advances and Challenges

Juliana Pereira Lopes Gonçalves, PhD, Christine Bollwein, MD,
Wilko Weichert, MD, Kristina Schwamborn, MD, PhD*

KEYWORDS

- Mass spectrometry imaging • Pathology • Histology • Clinical research
- Tissue imaging • Molecular imaging

KEY POINTS

- Mass spectrometry imaging (MSI) is a versatile technique capable of mapping the precise location of analyte molecules in tissue samples.
- MSI has been applied in different areas of histomorphological characterization of tumor lesions, such as biomarker identification, tumor diagnosis, and delineation of tumor margins.
- Reproducibility, validation, data analysis, and data storage are the main barriers to the establishment of the methodology in routine clinical care.

To treat any condition, the first step should be an unambiguous and precise diagnosis. Especially in cancer therapy, the diagnosis is essential to suggest the more appropriate course of treatment. In pathology, a myriad of tests and technologies is applied to assist a better diagnosis. However, there are still several tests that are ambiguous, time-consuming, and expensive. Some of those techniques resort to proteomics to unveil specific features of a heterogenic set of pathologies.

Because of its high sensitivity and specificity, mass spectrometry was granted the status of the method of choice for analysis of proteins, peptides, and metabolites. Mass spectrometry, in particular, liquid chromatography-mass spectrometry (LC-MS), has been introduced to identify proteomic derivatives that can elucidate the tumor microenvironment.[1] However, the limitations of this technique (low spatial resolution and heavy sample processing) are being overcome by mass spectrometry imaging (MSI).

Institute of Pathology, Technical University of Munich, Trogerstr. 18, 81675 Munich, Germany
* Corresponding author.
E-mail address: kschwamborn@tum.de

Clin Lab Med 41 (2021) 173–184
https://doi.org/10.1016/j.cll.2021.03.001
0272-2712/21/© 2021 Elsevier Inc. All rights reserved.

labmed.theclinics.com

MASS SPECTROMETRY IMAGING

MSI is a technique that combines sensitivity and precision of mass spectrometry with the spatial resolution of imaging microscopy. It is being used in different fields, like drug ADME studies and quantification of metabolites in a specific tissue. But some of the most promising applications of MSI are in pathology, as a support tool to pathologists in diagnosis, prognosis, and biomarker discovery.[2]

Technologies and Basic Principles

There are 3 main components in mass spectrometry instrumentation: the ionization source, the ion separation method, and detection (**Fig. 1**).

The ionization sources most commonly used in MSI are desorption electrospray ionization (DESI), matrix-assisted laser desorption/ionization (MALDI), and secondary ion mass spectrometry (SIMS). There are also other techniques used, such as laser ablation electrospray ionization (LAESI) and laser ablation-inductively coupled plasma (LA-ICP).[3,4]

In DESI, the sample is sprayed at a defined angle, with an electrically charged solvent mist that causes the sample to ionize. This technique requires the least sample preparation and is the least destructive; on the other hand, it has the lowest spatial resolution. This approach is applicable to liquid, solid, frozen, and gaseous samples.[4]

MALDI involves desorption and ionization of molecules by an ultraviolet laser; they are then directed to a detector. The ions are subjected to an electric field that helps to keep the charged state. This approach allows for the measurement of a wider mass range but has lower spatial resolution than SIMS. MALDI also requires the application of a chemical matrix, which can generate specific peaks or adducts in the mass spectra.[4]

In SIMS, the sample surface is bombarded with energetic particles of a plasma gas (sputtering), ejecting the ionized particles, which are then collected and analyzed. SIMS proves to be advantageous in providing the highest resolution. Despite requiring a long sample preparation time, this methodology is regarded as the most sensitive, capable of detecting analytes at very low concentrations.[3]

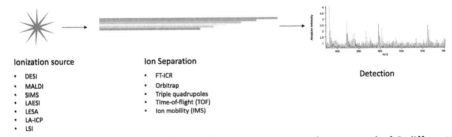

Ionization source
- DESI
- MALDI
- SIMS
- LAESI
- LESA
- LA-ICP
- LSI

Ion Separation
- FT-ICR
- Orbitrap
- Triple quadrupoles
- Time-of-flight (TOF)
- Ion mobility (IMS)

Detection

Fig. 1. Basic units of MSI technology. MSI apparatus commonly composed of 3 different parts: ionization source, ion separation, and detector. The choice of the machine is often correlated to the type of analyte that will be measured. After detection, the user gets 1 mass spectrum per ablated or sprayed region.

A significant limitation of MSI, especially compared with LC-MS, is the lack of separation prior to ionization. To retain spatial information, most common techniques require ablation of all ions in a pixel of the sample at the same time. This can lead to issues such as ion suppression. Nonetheless, to overcome this issue, postionization separation techniques have been developed. Most recently, ion mobility has been receiving a lot of interest for separation of analytes.[5,6] It has been seamlessly integrated into MALDI-MSI procedures. It has also been shown that it can be coupled with ambient ionization techniques (LAESI, LESA, and DESI). The technique allows the detection of specific classes and has shown an increase in the detected analytes.[7]

After ionization, analytes are separated based on their mass-to-charge ratio to generate a mass spectrum, which is acquired in the detector. Separation modules used include ion traps, Fourier-transform ion cyclotron resonance (FT-ICR), triple quadrupoles, orbitraps, and both axial and orthogonal acceleration time-of-flight (TOF) mass spectrometers.[5]

Furthermore, sample preparation depends on the type of instrument where the analysis will be carried out. For instance, in a MALDI on-tissue procedure, the sample is mounted on a conductive surface, followed by matrix layering. Depending on the analyte class and sample type, additional sample preparation steps such as enzymatic digestion or derivatization are also performed. The sample is then inserted in the mass spectrometer. Using a scanned image of the sample (**Fig. 2**A), the user defines the measurement regions. The defined resolution determines the area of the measurement spot (eg, 100 μm, 50 μm, or 10 μm). For those measurement spots, an individual

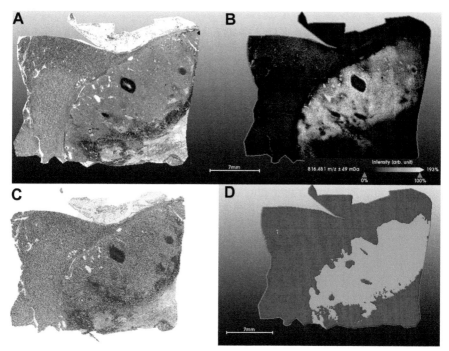

Fig. 2. Example of clear-cell renal cell carcinoma tissue section imaging analysis. (*A*) Initial slide scan used to define the measurement regions. (*B*) After mass spectrometry acquisition, it is possible to map the areas with higher and lower intensities for a defined m/z value (representation of m/z = 816,48 Da, possibly histone 2B fragment, using SCiLS laboratory software). (*C*) H&E scan used to define areas of interest to build new classifiers and for biomarker discovery. It can also be used to confirm results. (*D*) Bisecting k-means is a statistical tool capable of differentiating the tumor region from healthy tissue in a few seconds (representation using SCiLS laboratory software).

spectrum is recorded, and its specific position can, therefore, be precisely registered and correlated with the position in the scanned tissue. From the measurement of 1 sample, hundreds to thousands of spectra are generated, representing the spatial distribution of the different ions (**Fig. 2B**). Hence, the obtained data can be used to compare different samples or different regions in the same section (**Fig. 2C and D**). The large dataset collected represents a vast number of analytes (eg, peptides and metabolites) obtained in that specific tissue.

Different Mass Spectrometry Imaging Samples from Pathologic Tissues

Conveniently, MSI is versatile in its ability to accommodate different samples (blood, serum, fresh and frozen tissue, formalin-fixed paraffin-embedded [FFPE] tissue, cell culture, tissue microarrays, partial tissue sections, etc.), with different provenance of materials (tumor resection, core needle biopsy samples, organoids, cell-culture, etc.), and to analyze soluble extracted analytes from tissue samples. There is likewise versatility in the types of analytes that can be measured, including metabolites, proteins/peptides, glycans, and lipids. Such a variety of samples and analytes makes MSI an attractive approach for analysis in pathology. Moreover, sample preparation procedures often take into consideration that MSI can be easily integrated into clinical procedures.[8]

Samples can be quickly frozen (for structural integrity) and analyzed. In addition, after diagnosis, FFPE tissue sections are, per protocol, stored in pathology institutes, usually with well documented patient history, including treatment, disease progress, treatment response and survival.[9] From FFPE samples, it is possible to cut smaller sections of different parts of the tissue or different patient samples and build a new tissue microarray (TMA).[10] Hence, FFPE samples have been widely employed for MSI characterization. Protocols for preparation of FFPE samples have been developed and thoroughly studied, and consist of deparaffinization and antigen retrieval, followed by enzymatic digestion and, when required, matrix deposition.[9,11–13]

The previously mentioned capability of combining FFPE samples into TMAs is especially powerful to build new classifiers, because several smaller sections of samples from different patients/tumors are assembled and can be prepared and measured under the same experimental conditions. For the same reasons, TMAs are also frequently employed for high-throughput biomarker research.

Regardless of the sample measured, after the data acquisition, data processing and analysis are required. Overall, it is still a protracted process and in need of optimization to decrease the time from preparation to results.

MASS SPECTROMETRY IMAGING APPLICATIONS IN PATHOLOGY

The diagnosis of cancer is a procedure that entails several steps. Initially, the tumor family (eg, carcinoma, lymphoma, sarcoma, or melanoma) is determined. This is followed by a process to identify the tumor subentity, the cell/organ of origin, and the predictive biomarkers or druggable targets (eg, HER2, KRAS) in order to assist in the decision of the most appropriate therapy. This process can require considerable use of samples (collected tissue) and tests (immunohistochemical and genetic). Sometimes, when the sample is small, it is not possible to carry out all the essential tests for a meticulous assessment, simply because of the lack of tumor tissue in the specimen.[14]

Another task carried out by pathologists is to aid surgeons during the tumor resection, to help delimit the tumor margins.

The choice of the best treatment course is often based on the pathologists evaluation of prognostic biomarkers by characterization of morphomolecular composition of the tissue. Targeted therapeutics heavily rely on the presence of specific predictive molecular alterations.[2]

Taking into consideration the main activities in pathology for the diagnosis, evaluation, morphologic delimitation, specific biomarker identification, and prognosis prediction, it is expected that MSI can be of great support for a more objective molecular evaluation.

Herein the authors focus on the latest literature available that they consider relevant for the future clinical uses of MSI in pathology. Nonetheless, the authors recommend some manuscripts that sum up earlier efforts and further applications.[2,14]

Biomarker Discovery

Several efforts in the establishment of MSI as a tool for pathology have been directed to finding biomarkers that will help to objectively classify the tumor. Biomarker discovery has the purpose to find specific molecules or patterns in the sample that can help with tumor analysis and prognosis for targeted therapies. This approach allows for a specific and personalized diagnosis, which in turn will guide the chosen treatment.

Morse and colleagues[15] took a meaningful step toward prostate tumor diagnosis using MSI on needle core biopsies. By studying the metabolic profiles of prostate tissue, they identified 25 metabolites that behave distinctively in tumor and healthy tissue. Based on the significant differences, a multivariate classifier was built, achieving 85% accuracy on a test dataset and 96% accuracy on the training dataset.

In the field of skin lesions, MSI has also been shown to have a great potential. Margulis and colleagues[16] used 86 μm skin samples of basal cell carcinoma and normal tissue. The lipid and metabolites in the samples were measured by DESI-MSI, and statistical analysis, using a LASSO (least absolute shrinkage and selection operation) regression, identified 24 molecular ions relevant for tissue classification, which yielded an overall accuracy of 94.1%. Similar approaches can also be used to characterize tumor margins during intraoperative procedures, to ensure a complete resection of the tumor.

The potential of biomarker identification using MSI to complement established histopathological practice is summarized by Dilillo and colleagues.[17]

Tumor Diagnosis

Tumor diagnosis, usually performed by experienced pathologists, heavily relies on microscopic analysis and antigen testing. It can be challenging, however, to effectively discern the tissue sample for different reasons. The importance of an accurate and specific diagnosis cannot be emphasized enough, as it is the basis for deciding the patient's treatment course. Hence, 1 of the first studies of MSI on cancer was to find tumor diagnostic markers in contrast with healthy tissue.

In a recent study, 71 samples from patients with different subtypes of renal cell carcinoma, oncocytoma, and normal tissue were subjected to MSI measurement. Zhang and colleagues[18] applied a LASSO regression for discriminating between the different subtypes of renal cell carcinoma and normal tissues, which yielded a classification power of 100% per patient.

Fine needle aspiration is commonly used to assess malignancy of suspicious thyroid lesions. But to reliably distinguish between malignant and benign lesions can be difficult if not impossible when it concerns follicular lesions, frequently leading to diagnostic surgery, with most cases later receiving a benign diagnosis. DeHoog and colleagues used MSI analysis of 178 samples to determine molecular signatures for different thyroid lesions, building statistical classifiers for normal, benign follicular adenoma, and malignant follicular thyroid carcinoma and papillary thyroid carcinoma.[19] The accuracy of the classifiers was tested on 69 fine needle aspirations analyzed by MSI, yielding accuracies of 89% to 93%.

Sometimes tumors present similar histomorphological characteristics, which makes the diagnosis a challenging process. Also, to distinguish metastases from the primary tumor can be demanding, potentially resulting in a false classification of tumor stage and subsequently the wrong choice of treatment. In these cases, MSI analysis can be used to assist the pathologist in making a more accurate diagnosis.

Paine and colleagues used mouse models to study the lipid profiles of medulloblastomas.[20] The authors were able to identify patterns that indicate different tumor development stages. In the same study, they identified lipids, such as phosphatidylethanolamines, phosphatidic acids, phosphatidylserines, and phosphoinositides that are able to define the primary tumor boundaries as well as metastasis. This work, despite not being directly on human tissue, gives great insight into the metastatic process and may lead to the discovery of novel biomarkers for diagnosis and treatment of metastasizing medulloblastomas in humans.

Another research work on medulloblastoma and pineoblastoma, carried out by Clark and colleagues, evaluated the lipid content of frozen human samples by MSI.[21] Because both malignancies have similar histopathological characteristics, the researchers aimed to find a set of lipids that could better define each tumor. Based on their analysis, higher content of glycerophophoglycerols is indicative of medulloblastoma, while higher content of sphingolipids is associated with pineoblastoma.

Tumor staging is also an essential component of the diagnosis, which is important to determine how far the tumor has advanced. Briggs and colleagues studied the alterations on the fragmentation of N-glycans from epithelial ovarian cancer tissue using MSI and identified a set of staging biomarkers to successfully characterize early and late-stage tumors.[22]

Another study on protein N-glycosylation of epithelial ovarian cancer presented different N-glycans on early and late-stage tumor sections, further supporting the viability of MSI techniques to assist in tumor staging.[23]

Intraoperative Consultation

MSI not only has great potential in standard histopathological work-up but also offers the possibility to provide decisive support in the frozen section examination. This process, carried out in parallel with surgery, aims to avoid tumor regrowth by removing all the affected tissue, minimizing the damage to the tumor-adjacent tissue, thus ensuring the vital activity of the organ. There is a need for fast assessment of the resected sample, and MSI has great potential to assist in decision making.

There are some intraoperative surgical questions that currently cannot be answered accurately. An example of this is the limited differentiation between a primary carcinoma or the metastasis of a carcinoma located elsewhere, especially when dealing with a poorly differentiated carcinoma or when further clinical information is lacking (eg, primary mucinous neoplasm of the ovary vs ovarian metastasis of mucinous colorectal neoplasm[24,25] or primary adenocarcinoma/squamous cell carcinoma of the lung vs pulmonary metastasis of adenocarcinoma/squamous cell carcinoma of different location).[26] Another difficulty involves the detection of single-cell infiltrates or infiltrates of small tumor cell clusters (eg, infiltrates of lobular breast carcinoma in axillary sentinel lymph nodes).[27] These are scenarios in which surgical pathology can clearly benefit from MSI. Up to now, its application in frozen section analysis has been complicated because of protracted sample preparation and long measurement time. However, Basu and colleagues[13] introduced a modified procedure that allows sample processing in a total of 5 to 10 minutes using precoated slides, a high-frequency laser, and dimensionality reduction techniques. It is therefore within the normal timeframe of histologic processing for frozen section. A comprehensive review of MSI applications in cancer diagnosis and intraoperative consultation can be found elsewhere.[28]

Prognostic Predictors

New targeted therapeutic regimes rely heavily on predictive molecular variation within the patient's lesion. Such variations can help predict treatment outcome or how aggressive the tumor behaves.

When analyzing triple-negative breast cancer and correlating the results with Kaplan-Meier survival curves, Phillips and colleagues identified 9 peptide products derived from proteins, namely COL1A1, COL1A2, COL6A3, ATIC, CCDC24, PLEKHG2, SOX11, UBR4, and ZSWIM8, that correlated with prognosis.[29] For the first 8 peptides, high expression was associated with worse patient outcomes (P<.05). Moreover, COL1A1 and COL1A2, 2 components of type-I collagen, were shown to be upregulated in invasive breast cancer, with a potential role in spinal metastasis. Subtypes of collagen 1 are also upregulated in other tumor types such as metastatic ovarian cancer, cholangiocarcinoma, and other malignancies.

Ovarian high-grade serous carcinoma (HGSC) and borderline ovarian tumors (BOT) have different tumor invasion behaviors and different prognoses. Histopathology is used for diagnosis of serous ovarian cancer, but there is a therapeutic need for a more sensitive method that provides molecular information to better predict the tumor development. In a thorough study of serous ovarian cancer, Sans and colleagues[7] employed MSI to characterize molecular profiles of HGSC, BOT, and normal ovarian tissue samples. By statistical comparison of the metabolite and lipid profiles of the 3 different tissue types, the authors were able to identify a series of markers that helped predict the tumor aggressiveness and therefore the tumor subtype. For instance, while metabolite analysis revealed that in BOT nonoxidized forms of gluconic acid, hexose, and glucose could be found in higher abundance, N-acetylaspartic acid was determined to be a predictive feature of HGSC. Taurine and ascorbic acid were associated with healthy ovarian tissue, whereas negative modulation of succinate and malate were associated with tumor lesions.

Intratumor Heterogeneity

Intratumor heterogeneity is the result of the subclonal evolution of cancer cells within a tumor. This anomaly can be observed in many neoplasias and leads to different evolution regarding metastatic seeding and therapy resistance. In the same study on serous ovarian cancer, Sans and colleagues[7] found that MSI enables clear visualization of the papillary branches in serous BOT and characterization of tumor heterogeneity. For five different HGSC samples that contained clear stroma tissue adjacent to the tumor, a statistical classification between both tissue types yielded 99.5% accuracy when compared with annotations from a pathologist.

In another promising study exploring breast cancer heterogeneity, Alberts and colleagues[30] carried out a protein profiling of invasive ductal breast cancer using MALDI imaging. The sample data were processed by clustering to identify different sections in the tumor region and compared with histopathological annotations. Afterward, the various subsections were separated by laser microdissection, and the proteomic content was evaluated by liquid chromatography-tandem mass spectrometry (LC-MS/

MS). Proteins, such as Keratin type-I cytoskeletal 9, and Keratin type-II cytoskeletal 8 were found in different concentrations in different parts of the tumor.

These types of studies have immense potential to identify proteins in tissue sections and enable large-scale identification of biomarkers related to intratumor heterogeneity. Further revisions on the use of MSI for investigation of tumor heterogeneity are summarized elsewhere.[31]

CHALLENGES

As outlined previously, MSI offers versatile applications in pathology. There are, however, some issues that must be addressed before MSI can be established as an integral part of routine diagnostics.

Standardization and validation are crucial in diagnostic procedures. Standardized protocols have to encompass all steps, from sample preparation, instrumentation, and data analysis, so that a high level of reproducibility and repeatability can be ensured. In recent years, the awareness for the reproducibility of MSI has increased, and several studies have been conducted accordingly.[9] The largest study so far investigated tissue typing data based on tryptic peptides spectra of human and mouse FFPE material acquired at 5 different institutions.[32] By adhering to a comprehensive workflow, Ly and colleagues showed that it is not only possible to maintain high spectral resolution but also to ensure the acquisition of comparable data. Nevertheless, the authors emphasized that some degree of technical variance would always occur, although it would not prevent a correct classification. Contradictorily, the results presented by Buck and colleagues[33] on murine FFPE tissues across multiple centers are a reminder that further efforts are required to incorporate MSI in routine diagnostics. Focusing on peptide and metabolite data, they demonstrated that intracenter and intercenter technical variances were so marked as to have negative impacts on the performance of univariate classification, despite identical-to-similar technical equipment and sample preparation. In contrast, multivariate classification achieved much better values, especially when the classifier was built using data from several centers. This key finding highlights the importance of establishing data libraries that can be used as a basis for building, refining, and applying tissue classifiers as part of software development and data analysis.

There has been great progress in this field in recent years, with a plethora of data processing tools available today, ranging from open source to proprietary software. The large amount of data generated during a high spatial and mass resolution run poses a challenge in data processing.[34] Some approaches have been developed to overcome this issue, such as peak picking and dimensionality reduction algorithms.[35] Once a limited number of relevant biomarkers has been defined, it is expected that the required computing and memory capacity will decrease. Further focus on bioinformatics is directed toward quality control that is aimed at monitoring and solving reproducibility issues. Special methods and functions for this task have already been established in the form of open-source packages (MALDIrppa, R-package)[36] or as part of computational platforms (Galaxy).[37]

Accomplishing more reproducible studies, better classifiers, and user-friendly software will allow for the technology to be submitted for approval by the competent authorities like the US Food and Drug Administration or European Medicines Agency.

The points mentioned previously make it clear that the introduction of MSI in routine pathology still requires considerable effort. Additionally, to implement this methodology, medical divisions must consider the financial investment. This not only refers to the technical equipment (eg, mass spectrometry instrument or matrix sprayer) but also to the software packages needed for analysis and infrastructure for data management and storage. The major expense factor is of course the mass spectrometer itself. Nevertheless, experience in microbiology has shown that implementation of MALDI-TOF-MS in the long run results in savings compared with the current methods because of its low reagent costs. Tran and colleagues[38] calculated that the cost of their instrument would balance out after 3 years. Such long-term savings potential is also conceivable in pathology given the numerous supplementary tests, especially immunohistochemical staining, required for an accurate diagnosis. Complex and expensive molecular analyses could also be at least partially replaced by MSI as demonstrated by Bonaparte and colleagues on lung cancer specimens.[39]

EXPECTATIONS AND OUTLOOK

There are many important questions about MSI that remain to be answered:

Is it possible to discern aggressive tumors from nonaggressive tumors?
Can the efficacy of therapy be predicted before starting treatment?
Can a patient be treated by targeting solely the tumor without unnecessarily harming the patient?

Although there are still no simple answers to those questions, MSI has been proven to be useful in reaching a deeper knowledge about the histomolecular composition of tumors. In the most different fields of oncology, and especially as a supportive methodology in pathology, MSI has been asserting itself as a valuable resource. Unlike the current methods that offer standardized tests for the characterization of lesions, MSI offers a more personalized approach, as it analyzes the individual patient samples, looking for its biomarkers and prognostic predictors; thus a more tailored therapy could be applied. There are certainly some obstacles toward the standardization and accreditation of the technology. Some of the obstacles can be overcome by establishing a method of measurement and calibration using internal standards for every measurement. In addition, a universal and rapid sample preparation protocol that can be adopted in the diverse pathology units with comparable data acquired is also required for the success of the methodology. Before the technology leaps into the clinic, a software version that is, both user-friendly and that generates compressed data is also needed. The authors believe that a large database, such as METASPACE, where different MSI data can be deposited, can benefit the transition from research to routine laboratories.[40] This has the potential to not only help create more accurate classifiers, but especially for cases with challenging diagnosis and for identification of rarer tumor types. For these rarer tumor types, MSI data of a specific patient could be crosschecked with the database for a similar profile, helping diagnosis and consequent therapy.

As the authors see it, all present limitations can be solved in the near future with combined effort and further research.

CLINICS CARE POINTS

- MSI provides sensitive and precise information about the molecular landscape directly on tissue sections and can assist in biomarker discovery, intraoperative consultation, and evaluation of intratumor heterogeneity.
- MSI has been used for the analysis of metabolites, peptides/ proteins, glycans, and lipids in fresh frozen as well as FFPE tissue, cytology and cell culture samples.

- Fast and transversal protocols, as well as standardization and validation, have to be addressed before further advancement of the technology into clinical diagnostics.
- Data processing and analysis still present a bottleneck of MSI, where a plethora of approaches has been proposed, but insufficient effort has been directed to establishing a universal quality control method.
- MSI offers a personalized approach, as it has the potential to screen individual patient samples for its biomarkers and prognostic predictors without the need for target specific reagents such as antibodies.

ACKNOWLEGMENTS

The authors gratefully acknowledge the financial support of the Deustche Krebshilfe (German Cancer Aid) for the INTEGRATE-TN project (grant number: 70113450).

DISCLOSURE

The authors have nothing to disclose.

REFERENCES

1. Nguyen EV, et al. Proteomic profiling of human prostate cancer-associated fibroblasts (CAF) reveals LOXL2-dependent regulation of the tumor microenvironment. Mol Cell Proteomics 2019;18(7):1410–27.
2. Vaysse PM, Heeren RMA, Porta T, et al. Mass spectrometry imaging for clinical research – latest developments, applications, and current limitations. Analyst 2017;142(15):2690–712.
3. Anderton CR. Mass spectrometry imaging: methodology and applications, . Encyclopedia of Spectroscopy and Spectrometry. Third Edition. Cambridge, Massachusetts, USA: Academic Press; 2017. p. 719–27.
4. Buchberger AR, DeLaney K, Johnson J, et al. Mass spectrometry imaging: a review of emerging advancements and future insights. Anal Chem 2018;90(1): 240–65.
5. Snel MF. Ion mobility separation mass spectrometry imaging. Comprehensive analytical chemistry, vol. 83. Amsterdam: Elsevier; 2019. p. 237–57.
6. Soltwisch J, Heijs B, Koch A, et al. MALDI-2 on a trapped ion mobility quadrupole time-of-flight instrument for rapid mass spectrometry imaging and ion mobility separation of complex lipid profiles. Anal Chem 2020;19:8.
7. Sans M, et al. Metabolic markers and statistical prediction of serous ovarian cancer aggressiveness by ambient ionization mass spectrometry imaging. Cancer Res 2017;77(11):2903–13.
8. Ly A, et al. High-mass-resolution MALDI mass spectrometry imaging of metabolites from formalin-fixed paraffin-embedded tissue. Nat Protoc 2016;11(8): 1428–43.
9. Hermann J, et al. Sample preparation of formalin-fixed paraffin-embedded tissue sections for MALDI-mass spectrometry imaging. Anal Bioanal Chem 2020;412(6): 1263–75.
10. Casadonte R, Longuespée R, Kriegsmann J, et al. MALDI IMS and cancer tissue microarrays. In: Drake RR, McDonnell LA, editors. Advances in cancer research, vol. 134. Cambridge, Massachusetts, USA: Academic Press Inc; 2017. p. 173–200.

11. Welker M, Van Belkum A, Girard V, et al. An update on the routine application of MALDI-TOF MS in clinical microbiology. Expert Rev Proteomics 2019;16(8): 695–710.

12. Johnson J, Sharick JT, Skala MC, et al. Sample preparation strategies for high-throughput mass spectrometry imaging of primary tumor organoids. J Mass Spectrom 2020;55(4):e4452.

13. Basu SS, et al. Rapid MALDI mass spectrometry imaging for surgical pathology. Npj Precis Oncol 2019;3(1):1–5.

14. Schwamborn K. The importance of histology and pathology in mass spectrometry imaging. In: Advances in cancer research, vol. 134. Academic Press Inc; 2017. p. 1–26.

15. Morse N, et al. Reliable identification of prostate cancer using mass spectrometry metabolomic imaging in needle core biopsies. Lab Invest 2019;99(10):1561–71.

16. Margulis K, Chiou AS, Aasi SZ, et al. Distinguishing malignant from benign micro-scopic skin lesions using desorption electrospray ionization mass spectrometry imaging. Proc Natl Acad Sci U S A 2018;115(25):6347–52.

17. Dilillo M, Heijs B, McDonnell LA. Mass spectrometry imaging: how will it affect clinical research in the future? Expert Rev Proteomics 2018;15(9):709–16.

18. Zhang J, Li SQ, Lin JQ, et al. Mass spectrometry imaging enables discrimination of renal oncocytoma from renal cell cancer subtypes and normal kidney tissues. Cancer Res 2020;80(4):689–98.

19. DeHoog RJ, et al. Preoperative metabolic classification of thyroid nodules using mass spectrometry imaging of fine-needle aspiration biopsies. Proc Natl Acad Sci U S A 2019;116(43):21401–8.

20. Paine MRL, et al. Three-dimensional mass spectrometry imaging Identifies lipid markers of medulloblastoma metastasis. Sci Rep 2019;9(1):1–10.

21. Clark AR, et al. Rapid discrimination of pediatric brain tumors by mass spectrom-etry imaging. J Neurooncol 2018;140(2):269–79.

22. Briggs MT, et al. MALDI mass spectrometry imaging of early- and late-stage se-rous ovarian cancer tissue reveals stage-specific N-glycans. Proteomics 2019; 19:21–2.

23. Briggs MT, et al. MALDI mass spectrometry imaging of early- and late-stage se-rous ovarian cancer tissue reveals stage-specific N-glycans. Proteomics 2019; 19(21–22):e1800482.

24. Buza N. Frozen section diagnosis of ovarian epithelial tumors diagnostic pearls and pitfalls. Arch Pathol Lab Med 2019;143(1):47–64.

25. Akrivos N, Thomakos N, Sotiropoulou M, et al. Intraoperative consultation in ovarian pathology. Gynecol Obstet Invest 2010;70(3):193–199..

26. Sienko A, Allen TC, Zander DS, et al. Frozen section of lung specimens. Arch Pathol Lab Med 2005;129(12):1602–9.

27. Layfield DM, Agrawal A, Roche H, et al. Intraoperative assessment of sentinel lymph nodes in breast cancer. Br J Surg 2011;98(1):4–17.

28. Zhang J, Sans M, Garza KY, et al. Mass spectrometry technologies to ADVANCE care for cancer patients IN clinical and intraoperative use. Mass Spectrom Rev 2020;mas.21664. https://doi.org/10.1002/mas.21664.

29. Phillips L, Gill AJ, Baxter RC. Novel prognostic markers in triple-negative breast cancer discovered by MALDI-mass spectrometry imaging. Front Oncol 2019; 9:379.

30. Alberts D, et al. MALDI imaging-guided microproteomic analyses of heteroge-neous breast tumors-A Pilot study. Proteomics Clin Appl 2018;12(1):1700062.

31. Balluff B, Hanselmann M, Heeren RMA. Mass spectrometry imaging for the investigation of intratumor heterogeneity. In: Drake RR, McDonnell LA, editors. Advances in cancer research, vol. 134. Cambridge, Massachusetts, USA: Academic Press Inc; 2017. p. 201–30.

32. Ly A, et al. Site-to-site reproducibility and spatial resolution in MALDI–MSI of peptides from formalin-fixed paraffin-embedded samples. Proteomics Clin Appl 2019;13(1):1800029.

33. Buck A, et al. Round robin study of formalin-fixed paraffin-embedded tissues in mass spectrometry imaging. Anal Bioanal Chem 2018;410(23):5969–80.

34. Trede D, Kobarg JH, Oetjen J, et al. On the importance of mathematical methods for analysis of MALDI-imaging mass spectrometry data. J Integr Bioinformatics 2012;9(1):189.

35. Verbeeck N, Caprioli RM, Van de Plas R. Unsupervised machine learning for exploratory data analysis in imaging mass spectrometry. Mass Spectrom Rev 2020;39(3):245–91.

36. Palarea-Albaladejo J, McLean K, Wright F, et al. MALDIrppa: quality control and robust analysis for mass spectrometry data. Bioinformatics 2018;34(3):522–3.

37. Föll MC, et al. Accessible and reproducible mass spectrometry imaging data analysis in Galaxy. Gigascience 2019;8(12):1–12.

38. Tran A, Alby K, Kerr A, et al. Cost savings realized by implementation of routine microbiological identification by matrix-assisted laser desorption ionization-time of flight mass spectrometry. J Clin Microbiol 2015;53(8):2473–9.

39. Bonaparte E, et al. Molecular profiling of lung cancer specimens and liquid biopsies using MALDI-TOF mass spectrometry. Diagn Pathol 2018;13(1). https://doi.org/10.1186/s13000-017-0683-7.

40. Alexandrov T, et al. METASPACE: a community-populated knowledge base of spatial metabolomes in health and disease. bioRxiv 2019;539478. https://doi.org/10.1101/539478.

Breath-Based Diagnosis of Infectious Diseases
A Review of the Current Landscape

Chiranjit Ghosh, PhD[a,b,1], Armando Leon, MD[a,b,1],
Seena Koshy, PhD[a,b], Obadah Aloum, MBBS[a,b],
Yazan Al-Jabawi, MBBS[a,b], Nour Ismail, MD[a,b],
Zoe Freeman Weiss, MD[a,b,c], Sophia Koo, MD[a,b,d],*

KEYWORDS

- Diagnosis • Breath • Metabolites • Biomarker • Point-of-care • Noninvasive • VOC

KEY POINTS

- The most accurate existing diagnostic methods for infectious diseases are usually invasive, with limited sensitivity, and require specialized laboratories and techniques.
- There is a need for the development and implementation of noninvasive, point-of-care diagnostic tools for viral, parasitic, bacterial and fungal infections.
- Breath-based testing has already shown significant promise as an alternative to conventional diagnostic tools for rapid, real-time identification of various pathogens.
- Breath tests may also provide information about treatment response and thus guide antimicrobial therapy and reduce antimicrobial resistance.
- Technologies explored so far for breath analysis include: electronic nose sensor, GC-MS, GC-TOF-MS, PTR-SIFT-MS, IMS-DMS, SPME-GC-MS, and nanomaterial gas sensor.

INTRODUCTION

Breath has been proposed to hold diagnostic clues to pathophysiologic processes since ancient times. Ancient Greek physicians described a sweet smell in patients

Funded by: NIHHYB. *Grant number(s):* R01 AI138999; R21 AI130669; R21 AI133330; R21 AI156279; R44 AI141264. *NIHMS-ID:* 1680788.
[a] Division of Infectious Diseases, Brigham and Women's Hospital, 181 Longwood Avenue, MCP642, Boston, MA 02115, USA; [b] Harvard Medical School, 25 Shattuck Street, Boston, MA 02115, USA; [c] Division of Infectious Diseases, Massachusetts General Hospital, Boston, MA 02114, USA; [d] Dana-Farber Cancer Institute, 450 Brookline Avenue, Boston, MA 02215, USA
[1] These authors contributed equally to this work.
* Corresponding author. Division of Infectious Diseases, Brigham and Women's Hospital, 181 Longwood Avenue, MCP642, Boston, MA 02115.
E-mail address: skoo@bwh.harvard.edu

with diabetes and a fishlike odor emanating from patients with what is now known to be kidney disease.[1]

The modern era of breath analysis started when biochemist Linus Pauling characterized the landscape of volatile organic compounds (VOCs) in human breath using methods available to him at the time, finding these VOCs to originate from numerous endogenous biochemical processes, including aldehydes and alkanes from lipid oxidation and ketones from carbohydrate and fatty acid metabolism.[2–5] Gas-phase metabolites and breakdown products originating from these processes are carried through the circulatory system and rapidly excreted through the lungs.

These VOCs are diluted in a bulk matrix of nitrogen, oxygen, carbon dioxide, water vapor, and inert gases, and typically present in trace concentrations in the breath. Although a few highly abundant compounds, such as acetone, are present in the low parts-per-million range, most VOCs are present in the low parts-per-billion (ppb) to parts-per-trillion (ppt) range. The low concentration of these analytes is one of the challenges in reliably identifying metabolic changes in the breath that indicate disease processes, with the need for methods to concentrate these metabolites before analysis on most analytical instrumentation. Other challenges include the natural variability of breath compounds diurnally and with varying age and sex; the potential for exogenous VOCs from the patient's environment in the breath sample; the chemical complexity of breath samples, which can contain hundreds to a thousand VOCs; and the lack of standardized methods for breath collection, which in aggregate may lead to findings that are not generalizable.[6]

Furthermore, the term breath analysis is primarily used when referring to the analysis of VOCs, which are truly volatile or semivolatile and found in the gas phase of the breath sample, but it is also sometimes used to refer to the analysis of larger molecules, including nucleic acids and proteins, suspended in aerosols and droplets in the liquid component of the breath. To analyze this fraction of the breath, the breath is generally collected in a cooled container and the condensate examined for these analytes.

With the development of effective preconcentration methods and increasingly sensitive analytical instruments capable of identifying and quantifying analytes at ultra-trace levels, various analytes in the exhaled breath have been assessed for the identification of pathophysiologic processes, including infectious diseases. The ultimate objective of identifying and validating breath biomarkers of various infections is to identify these processes at an earlier stage than currently possible with existing culture, antigen, and molecular methods; to facilitate early, appropriate antimicrobial prescribing; to reduce unnecessary antimicrobial exposure; and to improve clinical outcomes in patients with these infections.

BREATH MATRICES

When searching for breath biomarkers in disease states, the breath matrix chosen for sampling plays a vital role in determining the type of information that can be obtained. Breath matrices are classified into 2 main phases: gaseous/volatile breath and breath condensate.[7] Most studies to date have been based on volatile breath, which contains low-molecular-weight volatile and semivolatile compounds.[8] VOCs in breath can originate from different sources, and their concentrations in the breath are caused by both endogenous (normal human metabolism, products of microbial metabolism in the oral cavity, lungs, or digestive system) and exogenous (environmental exposure occurring through inhalation, ingestion, or skin absorption of these VOCs) factors. Exhaled breath components originate either from alveolar breath or from dead-space air.

Alveolar breath comes from gas exchange in the lungs, whereas the sources of dead-space air, the volume of air that is inhaled but does not take part in gas exchange, include the mouth, trachea, and bronchi.

INSTRUMENTS FOR BREATH ANALYSIS
Gas Chromatography

After preconcentration of breath VOCs using sorbent materials, the most common technique used for chemical separation, detection, and measurement of these VOCs is gas chromatography (GC) coupled with a detector, such as a mass spectrometer or flame ion detector (FID).[9] After desorption of samples, the analytes are carried through a chromatographic column by an inert gas and separated according to the chemical properties of the column, which can have a polar, midpolar, or nonpolar coating. Polar columns separate analytes based on their polarity after their chemical interactions with the column coating, whereas nonpolar columns separate analytes based on their boiling points.

Gas Chromatography Flamed Ionization Detector

GC can also be paired with an FID, which has the advantages of being significantly lower in cost than a mass spectrometer but still able to quantify known analytes accurately, with several studies using this method to measure hydrocarbons and other VOCs in human breath.[9,10] In an FID, inert carrier gas transfers analytes from the GC column to the FID, where volatile organic analytes in the breath sample undergo combustion in the presence of hydrogen and zero air to produce ions and free electrons, which eventually provide the information about the targeted analytes. GC-FID can be more sensitive for quantitative analysis than GC-mass spectrometry (MS), although GC-FID cannot be used to identify biological molecules or provide qualitative data.

Gas Chromatography Mass Spectrometry

GC-MS is widely used in breath research, especially for identification and interpretation of VOCs present in human breath. Sample preparation is an integral part of this technique where breath compounds are preconcentrated in a suitable device before analysis by GC-MS. Solid-phase microextraction (SPME) is one of the most popular techniques for headspace and solvent-free extraction, using needlelike fibers with a sorbent coating.[11] However, SPME is limited to the extraction of hydrophilic compounds and is sometimes biased toward hydrophobic compounds in the breath. To overcome these limitations, sample preparation through sorbent trap devices has become a more widely used preconcentration method for VOCs.[12,13] GC-MS is based on the measurement of the mass-to-charge ratio (m/z) after analytes are fragmented by electron or chemical ionization, and the daughter ions are monitored for interpretation.[14–16] Large reference libraries, selection of predetermined run methods, and high sensitivity (in the ppt level when used in combination with preconcentration methods) for detection and quantification of breath compounds are the major advantages of this technique. However, the cost of GC-MS instruments and the need for regular operation and maintenance by highly skilled personnel have limited its widespread use in regular clinical settings.

Gas Chromatography Time-of-Flight Mass Spectrometry

For quantitative analysis of breath compounds, GC time-of-flight (TOF) MS has gained considerable popularity. In GC-TOF, ions are pulsed down a field-free flight tube, with smaller ions traveling faster than larger ions, with separation of analytes as they are registered on the detector. The primary advantage of GC-TOF is the ability to separate analytes quickly and also its high-resolution capability. Unlike scanning instruments, TOF-MS can acquire the chromatogram at a microsecond scale depending on the acquisition potential. GC-TOF-MS has been applied successfully to the detection of trace VOCs in the breath.[17–19]

Proton Transfer Reaction and Selected Ion Flow Tube Mass Spectrometry

Proton transfer reaction (PTR) MS and ion flow tube MS are potential platforms for on-line quantification of VOCs without any preconcentration. Both instruments rely on chemical ionization of the analytes. PTR-MS uses a soft ionization technique, where a specific reactant (generally H_3O^+) interacts through proton transfer with all analytes having an affinity for protons higher than water molecules.[20,21] After ionization, the molecules are accelerated through a drift tube after the application of a magnetic or electric field and passed to MS for analysis. In selected ion flow tube (SIFT) MS, ions are passed through a flow tube by a carrier gas in the presence of a small voltage to avoid possible diffusion to the walls of the tube.[22,23] Both instruments consist of a ion-generation zone, a reaction zone, and a detection zone.[24] The primary advantages of PTR-MS and SIFT-MS are the feasibility of fast analysis and high sensitivity, with the potential to measure VOCs from ppb to ppt levels.[25] However, both instruments are expensive and require regular maintenance by expert personnel.

Ion Mobility Spectrometry/Differential Mobility Spectrometry

Ion mobility spectrometry (IMS) and differential mobility spectrometry (DMS) are fast and sensitive analytical tools for the detection of a wide range of gas-phase molecules. These techniques were first used for the detection of chemical warfare agents in the atmosphere.[26] IMS/DMS can detect trace analytes in the ppb to ppt range. In IMS, ions are separated at ambient pressure in the presence of an external electric field.[27,28] The ions are transported to an electrode by a carrier gas and the drift time for ion swarm toward the electrode depends on the mobility of ions.[29] An electrical field is applied to the ions, and the ions reach the electrode at different times. IMS and DMS have the potential to provide online, rapid analysis of breath analytes. However, preconcentration is generally necessary, along with prior knowledge of target analytes to determine analyte levels.

Electronic Nose Sensor

The electronic nose (eg, eNose) is a simple device that can potentially be applied to breath analysis.[30] The eNose contains a sensor array that undergoes a physical change in response to a chemical input, and these changes are converted into electric signals, with a particular response to a chemical analyte or mixture of chemicals.[31,32] The signal produced by the eNose depends on the nature of the odor, the interaction of the chemical or chemical mixture with the sensors, and the type of sensors in the array.[33] Unlike laboratory-based benchtop instruments, eNoses are generally portable and do not require expensive components or skilled operators, with integrated neural network analyses being applied to discriminate the eNose signal from disease versus nondisease states. Although electronic noses are inexpensive and rapid, they are limited in their sensitivity and subject to blind spots, with alternative selective sensors sometimes being required for particular analytes.[34] The specific analytes that differentiate disease versus nondisease states cannot be identified using eNoses, so alternative detection techniques need to be used to identify and validate disease-specific biomarkers.

Nanomaterial Gas Sensors

Nanomaterial sensors have increasingly been investigated for breath VOC analysis, with the potential for inexpensive, point-of-care assessments.[35] The nanomaterials most commonly used in these gaseous nanosensors include single-walled carbon nanotubes (CNTs), nanowires of various materials, nanoporous chemioptical materials, and monolayer capped metal nanoparticles (MCNPs).[36,37] Nanoscale coating of sensor material provides a large surface area-to-volume ratio, facilitating trapping of VOCs in exhaled breath.[38,39] While designing nanomaterial gas sensors for clinical applications, it is necessary to tailor the sensor's dynamic range to VOC concentrations in the breath. The sensitivity of these sensors depends on their materials, because the optimal design of these nanomaterial sensors also requires prior knowledge of analyte targets.[40] A significant limitation of these nanomaterial sensors is that it is not possible to design a nanomaterial that captures the full range of volatile analytes that are biomarkers of disease states.

DIAGNOSTIC USES OF CLINICAL BREATH TESTS FOR INFECTIONS

The 2019 CDC Antibiotic Resistance Threats Report estimates 2.8 million infections caused by antibiotic-resistant (AR) pathogens, with 35,900 attributable deaths per year.[41] One primary driver for the selection of these AR organisms is the excessive use of empiric antimicrobial therapy, which is in turn driven by the low sensitivity of cultures and other microbiologic techniques in identifying certain infectious diseases accurately and rapidly. Considerable progress has been made over the past decade in the identification of VOC biomarkers associated with specific diseases, laying the groundwork for faster and earlier diagnosis of infections, with an increasing focus on determining optimal diagnostic cutoff values of analyte concentrations for this purpose.

    Some of the most relevant studies that have characterized breath analytes for the identification of specific infections are reviewed here.

Viral Infections

The ongoing coronavirus disease 2019 (COVID-19) pandemic has shown the need for widespread noninvasive, rapid, and accurate testing for screening and diagnosis to contain the spread of highly contagious viral infections. Unlike bacteria, fungi, or parasites, viruses do not have their own metabolism, instead using the host cell's metabolic machinery to replicate and spread, making it challenging to identify unique viral metabolites in the breath.

Severe acute respiratory syndrome coronavirus-2

Although rapid severe acute respiratory syndrome coronavirus-2 (SARS-CoV-2) viral reverse transcription polymerase chain reaction (RT-PCR) and antigen assays have come into widespread use over the past year, these assays still have diagnostic limitations and availability bottlenecks. To shorten testing time and make mass screening more feasible, breath-based VOCs analysis has been proposed as an alternative sampling and testing technique.[42] A recent study was performed to characterize metabolites in exhaled breath in adults undergoing invasive mechanical ventilation with severe COVID-19, compared with those with non–COVID-19 acute respiratory distress syndrome (ARDS).[43] The investigators concluded that breath VOCs, including methylpent-2-enal, 2,4-octadiene, 1-chloroheptane, and nonanal, may help distinguish patients with COVID-19 from those with non-COVID-19 ARDS. However, this study was limited by a small sample size (40 patients) and did not have an external validation cohort. Another study found that aldehydes (ethanal, octanal), ketones (acetone, butanone), and methanol were able to distinguish patients with COVID-19 from those with other conditions, including asthma, chronic obstructive pulmonary disease, bacterial pneumonia, and cardiac disease.[44] One recent pilot study examined the exhaled breath of 26 children with suspected SARS-CoV-2 infection, finding 6 VOCs (octanal, nonanal, heptanal, decane, tridecane, and 2-pentylfuran) to be significantly increased in infected patients compared with noninfected individuals. The sensitivity and specificity of this study were reported to be 100% and 66.6% respectively, although the sample size was small.[45] Jendrny and colleagues[46] performed another pilot study to characterize patients with COVID-19 through scent identification by dogs. They aimed to track the specific scent of SARS-CoV-2 infection and trained 18 dogs to discriminate saliva or tracheobronchial secretion samples from patients with SARS-CoV-2 versus samples from uninfected controls for 1 week. The dogs could identify the samples from patients with SARS-CoV-2 with an average diagnostic sensitivity of 82.63% and specificity of 96.35%, but with significant variability in performance between animals.[46] Ryan and colleagues[47] proposed exhaled breath condensate (EBC) as an alternative test sample for SARS-CoV-2 RT-PCR analysis to help reduce the false-negative testing rate of nasopharyngeal swab (NPS) samples. Although they reported enhanced sensitivity using the EBC sampling method (it detected the virus in 93.3% of negative NPS samples when using 4 gene targets [S/E/N/ORF1ab]), the sample size was small and the statistical significance of this difference could not be properly assessed.[47] Wintjens and colleagues[48] used a commercially available electronic nose (Aeonose, The Aeonose Company, Zutphen, Netherlands) for preoperative screening of 219 asymptomatic patients, and reported a sensitivity of 86% and a negative predictive value (NPV) of 96% for asymptomatic infection, although this work requires further validation.

Although promising, it is not clear whether these signatures are specific for SARS-CoV-2 or whether they represent generalizable metabolic changes from respiratory infections. This topic warrants further study.

Influenza A

Traxler and colleagues[49] obtained breath from swine infected with influenza A virus and observed that breath acetaldehyde, propanal, n-propyl acetate, methyl methacrylate, styrene, and 1,1-dipropoxypropane were increased during infection and declined after infection. They used needle trap microextraction coupled with GC-MS to differentiate infected and noninfected swine. Based on culture headspace extraction, the same group reported an increased level of n-propyl acetate in cells with viral infection compared with bacterial infection.[50] Purcaro and colleagues[51] performed culture headspace extraction from microliter plates seeded with human laryngeal cells (both for influenza A and respiratory syncytial virus [RSV]) and found compounds (for RSV, 2-methyl-pentane, methyl sulfone, 2,4-dimethyl-heptane, and 4-methyl-octane; for influenza A, acetone, n-hexane, and other unidentified molecules) that could effectively differentiate infected and uninfected cells, and also observed fluctuations related to the degree of infection. Another study used both headspace culture extraction and human breath analysis and reported that 2,8-dimethylundecane was decreased, and some alkanes present in exhaled breath were either increased or decreased after influenza vaccination.[52] The liquid phase of breath has also been investigated as a potential sample for influenza RNA testing. To determine the size of particles carrying respiratory viral RNA during coughing and breathing, Gralton and colleagues[53] monitored the exhaled breath of 53 patients with symptomatic respiratory viral infections and observed that they produce a range of particles carrying viral RNA when coughing and breathing.

Parasitic Infections

Although parasitology is one of the most neglected areas of infectious disease research, efforts have been made to identify breath profiles for some protozoans and helminths. The development of these assays might aid in the diagnosis of these neglected infections in areas with limited resources where they are most prevalent.

Malaria

A field study was performed in children with and without uncomplicated *Plasmodium falciparum* infection to assess the efficiency of a breath test to monitor natural human malaria by using thermal desorption-GC/MS. These investigators identified 6 VOCs (methyl undecane, dimethyl decane, trimethyl hexane, nonanal, isoprene, and tridecane) as potential markers of infection. They also observed that infection was correlated with the monoterpenes α-pinene and 3-carene in breath.[54] Another similar study, by Berna and colleagues,[55] concluded that concentrations of 9 compounds (carbon dioxide, isoprene, acetone, benzene, cyclohexanone, and 4 thioethers) varied significantly in individuals during the course of infection, with diurnal cyclical increase of thioethers in the breath with *P falciparum* but not with *Plasmodium vivax* infection. Further studies could focus on species-specific diagnosis, helping guide antimalarial treatment, and this technique could also be an effective tool to assess infection clearance.[56]

Cutaneous leishmaniasis

Welearegay and colleagues[57] used ligand-capped ultrapure metal (gold, copper, platinum) nanoparticle sensors for the detection of breath compounds of 28 Tunisian patients with cutaneous leishmaniasis and 32 healthy controls, followed by GC-MS analysis. They reported 96.4% sensitivity and 100% specificity for leishmaniasis with 9 potential biomarkers of infection: 2,2,4-trimethyl pentane, 4-methyl-2-ethyl-1-pentanol, methylvinyl ketone, nonane, 2,3,5-trimethyl hexane, hydroxy-2,4,6-trimethyl-5-(3-methyl-2 butenyl)cyclohexyl methylacetate, octane, 3-ethyl-3-methylheptane, and 2-methyl-6-methylene-octa-1,7-dien-3-ol. This study not only expands on the diagnosis of this neglected entity but also provides an encouraging example of the use of chemical sensors for accurate and early noninvasive detection of pathogens.[57]

Echinococcosis

Another promising study examined breath metabolites in 32 patients with cystic echinococcosis (CE) in Tunisia and 16 patients with alveolar echinococcosis (AE) in Poland, with 51 control patients enrolled at both study sites, finding a distinct profile for each subtype of this infection. Using GC-Q/TOF and ultrapure metal nanoparticle chemoresistive gas sensors for faster sample analysis, the investigators reported 75% sensitivity and 86.7% specificity for CE, 92.9% sensitivity and 88.9% specificity for AE, and 91.7% sensitivity and 92.7% specificity for distinguishing between CE and AE. They found 2 compounds, 1-tridecene and (E)-13-docosenoic acid, to be specific for CE and 7 compounds (hexadecane, heptadecane, eicosane, 11-(pentan-3-yl)henicosane, tetratriacontane, 2-methyloctacosane, hentriacontane) in AE. The investigators highlighted the potential of this test, especially using nanoparticle chemoresistive gas sensors, for population screening in remote areas.[58]

Bacterial Infections

It remains highly challenging to identify the specific microbial cause of bacterial pneumonia, despite its high incidence worldwide, and empiric antibiotic therapy remains the most common strategy in the clinical management of suspected bacterial pneumonia. Current diagnostic methods for bacterial pneumonia are highly limited in their sensitivity, in particular, and many patients with suspected bacterial pneumonia are treated with antibiotics without any diagnostic work-up.

A study by Rosón and colleagues[59] assessed 533 patients with community-acquired pneumonia (CAP) and found that only 39% were able to produce quality sputum samples, with sensitivity of only 57% for identification of *Streptococcus pneumoniae*. Another study, by Ewig and colleagues,[60] found sputum Gram stain and culture only useful in 24% of suspected CAP cases. Molecular analysis of sputum with techniques such as the rapid multiplex BioFire FilmArray Pneumonia Panel (FA-PP) show little incremental diagnostic sensitivity compared with culture, with a positive percentage agreement of 94.4% with standard respiratory cultures.[61] In addition, Garg and colleagues[62] described the spatial variations of bacteria within the lung in patients with cystic fibrosis, which raises even more questions about the reliability of respiratory samples. Because of these limitations in the sensitivity of existing diagnostic testing for CAP, breath-based testing for bacterial pneumonia is a potentially attractive alternative, with the relative simplicity of sample collection and ability to access microbial VOCs from within the airways and lung parenchyma.

Tuberculosis

A systematic review by Saktiawati and colleagues[63] examining 14 studies that used an electronic nose to diagnose pulmonary tuberculosis (TB) found a pooled sensitivity and specificity of 93%, but they also concluded that further development is needed to provide real-time results. It is also necessary to conduct studies in patients with culture-negative TB, where a breath test might have most utility, particularly in children. A study by Kolk and colleagues[64] in South Africa analyzed breath samples from 171 patients using GC-MS and found a sensitivity of 62% and specificity of 84% after a secondary validation. They found 7 compounds that discriminated breath samples of patients with TB and without TB and they were different from those produced in vitro by *Mycobacterium tuberculosis*. This finding led to the conclusion that these markers were potentially generated by the host response to TB rather than product of bacterial metabolisms.[64] Another study, by Phillips and colleagues,[65] also used GC-MS to test 226 high-risk symptomatic patients and reported 84% sensitivity, 64.7% specificity, and 85% accuracy for diagnosing active pulmonary TB overall. They reported a profile of active pulmonary TB that included the following 10 compounds: oxetane; 3-(1-methylethyl)-; dodecane, 4-methyl-; cyclohexane, hexyl-; bis-(3,5,5-trimethylhexyl) phthalate; benzene, 1,3,5-trimethyl-; decane, 3,7-dimethyl-, tridecane; 1-nonene 4,6,8-trimethyl-; heptane 5-ethyl-2-methyl; and 1-hexene, 4-methyl-. Both studies suggest that breath testing for TB might have a greater benefit when used for screening rather than diagnosis, although the study of TB VOC biomarkers in general suffers from a lack of reproducible biomarkers between individual studies.

A pilot study by Mellors and colleagues[66] reported 2 biomarkers [4-(1,1-dimethylpropyl)phenol and 4-ethyl-2,2,6,6-tetramethylheptane] that were not previously associated with *M tuberculosis* both in vitro and in the exhaled breath of 9 macaques, and they also described 38 breath compounds that discriminated between infected and uninfected macaques with an area under the curve (AUC) of 98%. The same group recently published another study with 31 pediatric subjects where they identified 4 compounds (decane, 4-methyloctane, and 2 unidentified analytes [A and B]) that differentiated 10 patients with confirmed TB (either by culture or Xpert MTB/RIF) from 10 patients without microbiological evidence of TB with a sensitivity of 80%

and a specificity of 100%. Patients with a high clinical suspicion of TB without positive microbiological confirmation of TB were excluded from these calculations; however, these 4 compounds were also found in their breath.[67]

McNerney and colleagues[68] validated an immunosensor and bio-optical breath analyzer device to detect the *M tuberculosis* antigen Ag85B in cough droplets in a field study. The proposed breath analyzer was able to detect this antigen in 23 of 31 (74%) patients with a specificity of 79%. Although a larger study would be needed for validation, this approach shows promise for diagnosis of culture-negative TB, which remains a significant unmet need.

Pseudomonas aeruginosa

Most studies in *Pseudomonas aeruginosa* infection have focused on the identification of respiratory tract colonization with this species. Purcaro and colleagues[69] collected the exhaled breath of mice in Tedlar sampling bags, with GC-TOF-MS analysis. They reported 9 metabolites (4 alkylated hydrocarbons, isoborneol, *p*-cymene, 2-hexanone, an alkylated alcohol, and an unknown compound) that could differentiate between infected and uninfected mice and 10 metabolites [2-hydroxyethyl acetate; 1,3-dimethylcyclopentanol; 2-methyl-2-butenal; (E)-, 4-cyclopentene-1,3-dione; aldehyde 1; alkylated hydrocarbon 5 and 6; cyclohexanol; and 2 methylated fatty acids] that could differentiate between strains of *P aeruginosa*. They used ultraviolet-killed and live *P aeruginosa* isolates and found that levels of 2-hexanone, among other compounds, were increased in mice infected with killed bacteria, and different compounds, including isoborneol, were increased in mice infected with live bacteria, the hypothesis being that the latter were the result of bacterial metabolism or the interaction of pathogen and murine host.[69] Suarez-Cuartin and colleagues[70] used electronic noses to differentiate patients with bronchiectasis with and without *P aeruginosa* respiratory tract colonization with 72% accuracy, and they were able to differentiate colonization by *P aeruginosa* from other colonizers (such as *Haemophilus influenzae*) with 89% accuracy. Robroeks and colleagues[71] characterized 14 VOCs via GC-TOF-MS in the breath of pediatric patients with cystic fibrosis, and identified with 100% accuracy the presence of airway colonization by *P aeruginosa*. Another study reported increased amounts of hydrogen cyanide (HCN) in the breath of children with cystic fibrosis and *P aeruginosa* colonization. High levels of breath HCN have been associated with *P aeruginosa* in vivo and in vitro.[72,73]

Rabis and colleagues[74] used multicapillary column IMS to examine the breath of 57 adult patients and found 21 signals that could differentiate patients colonized or infected with *P aeruginosa* from controls.

Staphylococcus aureus

A study in pediatric patients with cystic fibrosis was able to identify distinct VOC profiles (9 compounds), some increased in infected patients (1,4-pentadiene, ethanol, acetone, 2-butanone, undecane, 2-methyl-naphthalene) and some decreased (3-hydroxy-2-butanone, hexanal, isopropyl myristate) using GC-MS, which differentiated patients with and without *Staphylococcus aureus* airway infection with 100% sensitivity and 80% specificity. This study was limited by a small sample size, with only 18 patients in total, so further evaluation in a larger cohort is necessary.[75] Zhu and colleagues[76] studied *S aureus* and *P aeruginosa* pneumonia murine models for a 120-hour period using secondary electrospray ionization MS with partial least-squares discriminant analysis and described the infection breathprint pattern at 6 time points, rather than determining specific volatile compounds (similar to the electronic nose approach). They found changes in these breathprints predictive of time to clearance of infection between subjects, which they suggested might be used to predict the course of infections in humans and guide antimicrobial prescribing practices. They also concluded that examining breath signatures overall, rather than focusing on specific metabolites, might provide a fuller picture of the interaction between bacterial and host metabolites and mitigate the effect of intersubject variation.[76]

Streptococcus pneumoniae
van Oort and colleagues[77] performed intratracheal inoculation of male adult rats with *S pneumoniae* or *P aeruginosa* in conjunction with controls treated with saline. They then performed mechanical ventilation 24 hours later to extract breath VOCs and analyzed these compounds using GC-MS and SIFT-MS. In their GC-MS results, they found 8 compounds that could discriminate between infected and noninfected animals (4-methyloctane; octane, 2-5-dimethyl; tetrachlorethylene; an unidentified naphthalene compound; 2 unidentified cyclic compounds; an unidentified branched aldehyde; and another unidentified compound) with an receiver operating characteristic (ROC) AUC of 0.93; 14 compounds could differentiate between *S pneumoniae* and controls (octane, 4-methyl-; octane, 2,5-dimethyl; hexadecane, hexane, 2-,4-dimethyl-; 2-propanol, 1-methyloxy-; nonane, 2-methyl-; heptane, 2-,4-dimethyl-; 2 unidentified cyclic compounds; an unidentified naphthalene compound; and 4 other unidentified compounds) with an ROC AUC of 0.93; 3 compounds could distinguish *P aeruginosa* from controls (2-propenoic acid, 2-ethylhexyl ester; unidentified branched aldehyde; and an unidentified cyclic compound) with an ROC AUC of 0.98, and the ROC AUC for *S pneumoniae* versus *P aeruginosa* was 0.99. GC-MS proved to be more accurate for discrimination than SIFT-MS. These results support the potential for establishing species-specific bacterial profiles in bacterial pneumonia.[77]

Helicobacter pylori
After alcohol breathalyzer tests, the urea breath test for *Helicobacter pylori* infection is probably the most commonly used breath test, although this assay requires administration of exogenous ^{13}C-labeled urea. *H pylori* in patients infected with this bacterium hydrolyzes the ^{13}C-labeled urea into CO_2 and ammonia, with the labeled CO_2 being exhaled through the lungs and detected in the breath. This test not only helps diagnose *H pylori* infection but can also assess the response to treatment.[78] A study by Maity and colleagues[79] developed a point-of-care and cost-effective residual gas analyzer MS-based sensor coupled with a high vacuum chamber to detect *H pylori* from human breath in real time. They reported a 100% sensitivity and 93% specificity with positive predictive value and NPV of 95% and 100%, respectively, compared with biopsy *H pylori* assessment in 35 patients.[79] A study by Ulanowska and colleagues[12] used SPME-GC/MS to identify compounds such as 2-butanone, isobutane, and ethyl acetate that differentiated patients with *H pylori* from healthy controls.

Acinetobacter baumannii
One of the biggest challenges in identifying bacterial pneumonia is differentiating airway colonization from active infection. Gao and colleagues[80] studied 20 patients with *Acinetobacter baumannii* ventilator-associated pneumonia (VAP), 20 patients with *A baumannii* airway colonization, and 20 ventilated patients with no *A baumannii* in their respiratory tracts, and identified 8 compounds (1-undecene; nonanal; decanal; 2,6,10-trimethyldodecane; 5-methyl-5-propyl-nonane; longifolene; tetradecane; and 2-butyl-1-octanol) that discriminated between active infection and colonization.[80] Only 4 of these compounds (1-undecene, decanal, longifolene, tetradecane) matched their previous in vitro culture results, which supports the findings by Zhu and colleagues,[81] who reported only 25% to 34% of shared peaks between in vivo and

in vitro samples, suggesting a significant metabolic shift between bacterial growth in media and bacterial growth in the lung milieu.

Ventilator-associated pneumonia

A commercially available electronic nose was assessed for the diagnosis of VAP.[82,83] Using computed tomography scans as part of the reference standard, these studies reported a low level of accuracy ($\sim$60%) for discriminating patients with and without VAP. A pilot study by Filipiak and colleagues[84] found some compounds to overlap between the headspace gas of cultured swabs and the breath of patients infected with these bacteria. The presence of dimethyl sulfate was associated with non–species-specific emerging infection. This study was also able to identify markers associated with pathogen-derived metabolites in 22 ventilated patients. The presence of multiple coinfections and the small sample size did not allow full characterization of a profile for each bacterial species in vivo, but they did report some specific compounds such as 3-methyl-1-butene for *H influenzae*, 1-undecene for *P aeruginosa*, propene and butane for *S aureus* (also showing decreased levels after treatment), and acetonitrile and 2-pentanone for *Escherichia coli*.

Fowler and colleagues[85] examined a wide range of breath VOCs present in lower respiratory tract infections and concluded that the host inflammatory response might influence breath VOCs. Another study identified 1-propanol as a potential marker to track general bacterial growth in patients with pneumonia.[86] Some of these identified VOCs are potentially products of bacterial metabolic pathways and may be viable markers for screening of patients with suspected VAP.[87]

Acute appendicitis

Andrews and colleagues[88] studied breath samples from 53 patients in a surgical unit with suspected acute appendicitis using ion-molecule reaction MS and found significant differences in the concentration of acetone, isopropanol, propanol, butyric acid, and other unidentified compounds with m/z ratio of 56, 61, and 87 in patients with proven acute appendicitis compared with patients without appendicitis.

Fungal Infections

Fungal infections are a major cause of significant morbidity and mortality, particularly in immunocompromised patients. The diagnosis of these infections is often delayed because of the nonspecific symptoms of invasive fungal disease, limited sensitivity of respiratory tract and blood cultures and fungal antigen tests, and the general debilitation of immunocompromised patients, which makes definitive invasive biopsy procedures challenging.[89] Because of the difficulty of diagnosing these infections, mortality caused by invasive fungal disease remains very high despite the availability of a wide range of highly potent antifungal drugs.[90] More sensitive, rapid, and noninvasive tests would have a major impact on the management of patients with suspected invasive fungal disease.

Invasive aspergillosis

Aspergillus species are ubiquitously distributed in the environment and have virulence factors that make invasive aspergillosis (IA) the most common invasive mold infection in immunocompromised patients and a common cause of morbidity in patients with chronic lung disease. *Aspergillus fumigatus* has been described to produce 2-pentyl-furan when it is cultured on blood agar and nutrient agar medium. Based on this observation, one group analyzed breath from healthy subjects, patients receiving chemotherapy, and adults colonized or infected with *A fumigatus* with underlying comorbidities such as bronchiectasis, cystic fibrosis, or immunosuppression. The investigators reported that detection of 2-pentylfuran was able to detect *A fumigatus* in the airways with moderate sensitivity (77%) and specificity (78%).[91] However, further studies have not found 2-pentylfuran to discriminate breath samples from patients with and without *A fumigatus* infection. Koo and colleagues[92] characterized the breath volatile metabolic profile of *A fumigatus* and other *Aspergillus* species in vitro and in the breath of 64 patients with suspected IA using thermal desorption GC-MS. They identified a signature of sesquiterpene compounds including α-trans-bergamotene, β-trans-bergamotene, a β-vatirenene–like sesquiterpene, and transgeranylacetone that could identify patients with IA with 94% sensitivity and 93% specificity. A study using an electronic nose suggested a distinct VOC profile in the breath of patients with prolonged chemotherapy-induced neutropenia with IA versus controls.[93] This group also found that *A fumigatus* respiratory tract colonization could be determined with 89% accuracy in patients with cystic fibrosis using this electronic nose.[94]

Oral candidiasis
Hertel and colleagues[95] collected breath samples from 10 patients with oral candidiasis and 10 controls and found no correlation with the compounds that have been described in vitro in cultures of *Candida* spp. These investigators did not find a specific volatile profile in oral candidiasis, but found that compounds such as methyl acetate, 2-methyl-2-butanol, hexanal, and longifolene declined with antifungal therapy and that other compounds, such as 1-heptene, acetophenone, 3-methyl-1-butanol, decane, and chlorbenzene, increased after treatment in some patients.

SUMMARY

Breath analysis has the potential to improve the identification of pathophysiologic processes, especially infectious diseases, because microbes have many unique metabolic pathways that are distinct from human metabolism. Although there are many technical challenges in the rigorous identification and validation of breath biomarkers that distinguish patients with and without these infections, breath remains a particularly attractive matrix because of the noninvasive nature of sample collection and the ability to assess microbial processes that are particularly challenging to identify with standard culture, antigen, and molecular amplification-based approaches, especially infections that are predominantly based in the lung. With the recent development of increasingly sensitive analytical instruments and point-of-care technologies capable of identifying and quantifying volatile analytes at ultratrace levels and with further delineation of biomarker signatures that accurately identify patients with specific infectious disease syndromes, breath-based assays for these infections are highly likely to be adopted in clinical settings over the next decade. These breath-based assays will offer noninvasive, rapid, real-time identification of specific infections earlier than possible with current methods, in turn facilitating early, appropriate antimicrobial prescribing, reducing unnecessary antimicrobial exposure, and ultimately improving clinical outcomes in patients with these infections.

CLINICS CARE POINTS

- Breath tests for pulmonary tuberculosis may be more useful for screening than diagnosis.
- Breath tests for *Pseudomonas aeruginosa* and *Acinetobacter baumannii* have shown different metabolites in colonization vs infection.

- Specific sesquiterpene compounds have been characterized for the diagnosis of invasive aspergillosis.
- There is a variable and inconsistent correlation between metabolites extracted in vitro and those obtained in vivo.
- Although very promising, most published studies of breath-based diagnostics have small sample sizes with specific patient populations so generalizability is still a major issue.

REFERENCES

1. Amann A, Costello BL, Miekisch W, et al. The human volatilome: volatile organic compounds (VOCs) in exhaled breath, skin emanations, urine, feces and saliva. J Breath Res 2014;8(3):034001.
2. Pauling L, Robinson AB, Teranishi R, et al. Quantitative analysis of urine vapor and breath by gas-liquid partition chromatography. Proc Natl Acad Sci U S A 1971;68(10):2374–6.
3. Teranishi R, Mon TR, Robinson AB, et al. Gas chromatography of volatiles from breath and urine. Anal Chem 1972;44(1):18–20.
4. Frank H, Hintze T, Bimboes D, et al. Monitoring lipid peroxidation by breath analysis: endogenous hydrocarbons and their metabolic elimination. Toxicol Appl Pharmacol 1980;56(3):337–44.
5. Das S, Pal M. Review—non-invasive monitoring of human health by exhaled breath analysis: a comprehensive review. J Electrochem Soc 2020;167(3):037562.
6. Xu M, Tang Z, Duan Y, et al. GC-based techniques for breath analysis: current status, challenges, and prospects. Crit Rev Anal Chem 2016;46(4):291–304.
7. Hunt J. Exhaled breath condensate: an overview. Immunol Allergy Clin North Am 2007;27(4):587–96.
8. Kubáň P, Foret F. Exhaled breath condensate: determination of non-volatile compounds and their potential for clinical diagnosis and monitoring. A review. Anal Chim Acta 2013;805:1–18.
9. Mendis S, Sobotka PA, Euler DE. Pentane and isoprene in expired air from humans: gas-chromatographic analysis of single breath. Clin Chem 1994;40(8):1485–8.
10. Frank Kneepkens CM, Lepage G, Roy CC. The potential of the hydrocarbon breath test as a measure of lipid peroxidation. Free Radic Biol Med 1994;17(2):127–60.
11. Poli D, Goldoni M, Corradi M, et al. Determination of aldehydes in exhaled breath of patients with lung cancer by means of on-fiber-derivatisation SPME–GC/MS. J Chromatogr B 2010;878(27):2643–51.
12. Ulanowska A, Kowalkowski T, Hrynkiewicz K, et al. Determination of volatile organic compounds in human breath for Helicobacter pylori detection by SPME-GC/MS. Biomed Chromatogr 2011;25(3):391–7.
13. Martin AN, Farquar GR, Jones AD, et al. Human breath analysis: methods for sample collection and reduction of localized background effects. Anal Bioanal Chem 2010;396(2):739–50.
14. Beale DJ, Pinu FR, Kouremenos KA, et al. Review of recent developments in GC–MS approaches to metabolomics-based research. Metabolomics 2018;14(11):152.

15. Baldwin S, Bristow T, Ray A, et al. Applicability of gas chromatography/quadrupole-Orbitrap mass spectrometry in support of pharmaceutical research and development. Rapid Commun Mass Spectrom 2016;30(7):873–80.

16. Beckner Whitener ME, Stanstrup J, Panzeri V, et al. Untangling the wine metabolome by combining untargeted SPME–GCxGC-TOF-MS and sensory analysis to profile Sauvignon blanc co-fermented with seven different yeasts. Metabolomics 2016;12(3):53.

17. Williamson LN, Bartlett MG. Quantitative gas chromatography/time-of-flight mass spectrometry: a review. Biomed Chromatogr 2007;21(7):664–9.

18. Vreuls RJJ, Dallüge J, Brinkman UAT. Gas chromatography–time-of-flight mass spectrometry for sensitive determination of organic microcontaminants. J Microcolumn Sep 1999;11(9):663–75.

19. Ryan D, Watkins P, Smith J, et al. Analysis of methoxypyrazines in wine using headspace solid phase microextraction with isotope dilution and comprehensive two-dimensional gas chromatography. J Sep Sci 2005;28(9–10):1075–82.

20. Schwoebel H, Schubert R, Sklorz M, et al. Phase-resolved real-time breath analysis during exercise by means of smart processing of PTR-MS data. Anal Bioanal Chem 2011;401(7):2079–91.

21. Herbig J, Müller M, Schallhart S, et al. On-line breath analysis with PTR-TOF. J Breath Res 2009;3(2):027004.

22. Španěl P, Smith D. Selected ion flow tube: a technique for quantitative trace gas analysis of air and breath. Med Biol Eng Comput 1996;34(6):409–19.

23. Kharitonov SA, Yates D, Barnes PJ. Increased nitric oxide in exhaled air of normal human subjects with upper respiratory tract infections. Eur Respir J 1995;8(2):295–7.

24. Smith D, Španěl P. Application of ion chemistry and the SIFT technique to the quantitative analysis of trace gases in air and on breath. Int Rev Phys Chem 1996;15(1):231–71.

25. Schwarz K, Pizzini A, Arendacká B, et al. Breath acetone—aspects of normal physiology related to age and gender as determined in a PTR-MS study. J Breath Res 2009;3(2):027003.

26. Ewing RG. Ion mobility spectrometry, 2nd Edition by Gary A. Eiceman (New Mexico State University, Las cruces, NM) and Zeev Karpas (Nuclear Research Center, Beer-Sheva, Israel). CRC press (an imprint of Taylor and Francis group): Boca Raton, FL. 2005. XVI + 350. J Am Chem Soc 2006;128(16):5585–6.

27. Reynolds JC, Blackburn GJ, Guallar-Hoyas C, et al. Detection of volatile organic compounds in breath using thermal desorption electrospray ionization-ion mobility-mass spectrometry. Anal Chem 2010;82(5):2139–44.

28. Baumbach JI, Eiceman GA. Ion mobility spectrometry: arriving on site and moving beyond a low profile. Appl Spectrosc 1999;53(9):338A–55A.

29. Borsdorf H, Eiceman GA. Ion mobility spectrometry: principles and applications. Appl Spectrosc Rev 2006;41(4):323–75.

30. Farraia MV, Cavaleiro Rufo J, Paciência I, et al. The electronic nose technology in clinical diagnosis: a systematic review. Porto Biomed J 2019;4(4):e42.

31. Gardner JW, Bartlett PN. A brief history of electronic noses. Sens Actuators B Chem 1994;18(1–3):210–1.

32. Van Berkel JJBN, Dallinga JW, Möller GM, et al. A profile of volatile organic compounds in breath discriminates COPD patients from controls. Respir Med 2010;104(4):557–63.

33. Dragonieri S, Annema JT, Schot R, et al. An electronic nose in the discrimination of patients with non-small cell lung cancer and COPD. Lung Cancer 2009;64(2): 166–70.
34. Bos LD, Sterk PJ, Fowler SJ. Breathomics in the setting of asthma and chronic obstructive pulmonary disease. J Allergy Clin Immunol 2016;138(4):970–6.
35. Boots AW, van Berkel JJBN, Dallinga JW, et al. The versatile use of exhaled volatile organic compounds in human health and disease. J Breath Res 2012;6(2): 027108.
36. Broza YY, Haick H. Nanomaterial-based sensors for detection of disease by volatile organic compounds. Nanomedicine 2013;8(5):785–806.
37. Konvalina G, Haick H. Sensors for breath testing: from nanomaterials to comprehensive disease detection. Acc Chem Res 2014;47(1):66–76.
38. Dovgolevsky E, Tisch U, Haick H. Chemically sensitive resistors based on monolayer-capped cubic nanoparticles: towards configurable nanoporous sensors. Small 2009;5(10):1158–61.
39. Paska Y, Stelzner T, Christiansen S, et al. Enhanced sensing of Nonpolar volatile organic compounds by silicon nanowire field effect transistors. ACS Nano 2011; 5(7):5620–6.
40. Long Z, Kou L, Sepaniak MJ, et al. Recent advances in gas phase microcantilever-based sensing. Rev Anal Chem 2013;32(2).
41. Kadri SS. Key takeaways from the U.S. CDC's 2019 antibiotic resistance threats report for frontline providers. Crit Care Med 2020;48(7):939–45.
42. Walker HJ, Burrell MM. Could breath analysis by MS could be a solution to rapid, non-invasive testing for COVID-19? Bioanalysis 2020;12(17):1213–7.
43. Grassin-Delyle S, Roquencourt C, Moine P, et al. Metabolomics of exhaled breath in critically ill COVID-19 patients: a pilot study. EBioMedicine 2021;63:103154.
44. Ruszkiewicz DM, Sanders D, O'Brien R, et al. Diagnosis of COVID-19 by analysis of breath with gas chromatography-ion mobility spectrometry - a feasibility study. EClinicalMedicine 2020;29:100609.
45. Berna AZ, Akaho EH, Harris RM, et al. Breath biomarkers of pediatric SARS-CoV-2 infection: a pilot study. medRxiv 2020;2020.
46. Jendrny P, Schulz C, Twele F, et al. Scent dog identification of samples from COVID-19 patients – a pilot study. BMC Infect Dis 2020;20(1):536.
47. Ryan DJ, Toomey S, Madden SF, et al. Use of exhaled breath condensate (EBC) in the diagnosis of SARS-COV-2 (COVID-19). Thorax 2021;76(1):86–8.
48. Wintjens AGWE, Hintzen KFH, Engelen SME, et al. Applying the electronic nose for pre-operative SARS-CoV-2 screening. Surg Endosc 2020;1–8.
49. Traxler S, Bischoff A-C, Saß R, et al. VOC breath profile in spontaneously breathing awake swine during Influenza A infection. Sci Rep 2018;8(1):14857.
50. Traxler S, Barkowsky G, Saß R, et al. Volatile scents of influenza A and S. pyogenes (co-)infected cells. Sci Rep 2019;9(1):18894.
51. Purcaro G, Rees CA, Wieland-Alter WF, et al. Volatile fingerprinting of human respiratory viruses from cell culture. J Breath Res 2018;12(2):026015.
52. Phillips M, Cataneo RN, Chaturvedi A, et al. Effect of influenza vaccination on oxidative stress products in breath. J Breath Res 2010;4(2):026001.
53. Gralton J, Tovey ER, McLaws M-L, et al. Respiratory virus RNA is detectable in airborne and droplet particles. J Med Virol 2013;85(12):2151–9.
54. Schaber CL, Katta N, Bollinger LB, et al. Breathprinting reveals malaria-associated biomarkers and mosquito attractants. J Infect Dis 2018;217(10): 1553–60.

55. Berna AZ, McCarthy JS, Wang RX, et al. Analysis of breath specimens for bio-markers of Plasmodium falciparum infection. J Infect Dis 2015;212(7):1120–8.

56. Berna AZ, McCarthy JS, Wang XR, et al. Diurnal variation in expired breath vol-atiles in malaria-infected and healthy volunteers. J Breath Res 2018;12(4):46014.

57. Welearegay TG, Diouani MF, Österlund L, et al. Ligand-capped ultrapure metal nanoparticle sensors for the detection of cutaneous leishmaniasis disease in exhaled breath. ACS Sensors 2018;3(12):2532–40.

58. Welearegay TG, Diouani MF, Österlund L, et al. Diagnosis of human echinococ-cosis via exhaled breath analysis: a promise for rapid diagnosis of infectious dis-eases caused by Helminths. J Infect Dis 2019;219(1):101–9.

59. Rosón B, Carratalà J, Verdaguer R, et al. Prospective study of the usefulness of sputum Gram stain in the initial approach to community-acquired pneumonia requiring hospitalization. Clin Infect Dis 2000;31(4):869–74.

60. Ewig S, Schlochtermeier M, Göke N, et al. Applying sputum as a diagnostic tool in pneumonia: limited yield, minimal impact on treatment decisions. Chest 2002; 121(5):1486–92.

61. Gastli N, Loubinoux J, Daragon M, et al. Multicentric evaluation of BioFire FilmAr-ray Pneumonia Panel for rapid bacteriological documentation of pneumonia. Clin Microbiol Infect 2020.

62. Garg N, Wang M, Hyde E, et al. Three-Dimensional microbiome and metabolome cartography of a diseased human lung. Cell Host Microbe 2017;22(5):705–16.e4.

63. Saktiawati AMI, Putera DD, Setyawan A, et al. Diagnosis of tuberculosis through breath test: a systematic review. EBioMedicine 2019;46:202–14.

64. Kolk AHJ, van Berkel JJBN, Claassens MM, et al. Breath analysis as a potential diagnostic tool for tuberculosis. Int J Tuberc Lung Dis 2012;16(6):777–82.

65. Phillips M, Basa-Dalay V, Bothamley G, et al. Breath biomarkers of active pulmo-nary tuberculosis. Tuberculosis 2010;90(2):145–51.

66. Mellors TR, Nasir M, Franchina FA, et al. Identification of Mycobacterium tubercu-losis using volatile biomarkers in culture and exhaled breath. J Breath Res 2018; 13(1):16004.

67. Bobak CA, Kang L, Workman L, et al. Breath can discriminate tuberculosis from other lower respiratory illness in children. Sci Rep 2021;11(1):2704.

68. McNerney R, Wondafrash BA, Amena K, et al. Field test of a novel detection de-vice for Mycobacterium tuberculosis antigen in cough. BMC Infect Dis 2010; 10(1):161.

69. Purcaro G, Nasir M, Franchina FA, et al. Breath metabolome of mice infected with Pseudomonas aeruginosa. Metabolomics 2019;15(1):10.

70. Suarez-Cuartin G, Giner J, Merino JL, et al. Identification of Pseudomonas aeru-ginosa and airway bacterial colonization by an electronic nose in bronchiectasis. Respir Med 2018;136:111–7.

71. Robroeks CM, van Berkel JJBN, Dallinga JW, et al. Metabolomics of volatile organic compounds in cystic fibrosis patients and controls. Pediatr Res 2010; 68(1):75–80.

72. Enderby B, Smith D, Carroll W, et al. Hydrogen cyanide as a biomarker for Pseu-domonas aeruginosa in the breath of children with cystic fibrosis. Pediatr Pulmo-nol 2009;44(2):142–7.

73. Smith D, Spaněl P, Gilchrist FJ, et al. Hydrogen cyanide, a volatile biomarker of Pseudomonas aeruginosa infection. J Breath Res 2013;7(4):44001.

74. Rabis T, Sommerwerck U, Anhenn O, et al. Detection of infectious agents in the airways by ion mobility spectrometry of exhaled breath. Int J Ion Mobil Spectrom 2011;14(4):187–95.

75. Neerincx AH, Geurts BP, van Loon J, et al. Detection of Staphylococcus aureus in cystic fibrosis patients using breath VOC profiles. J Breath Res 2016;10(4): 46014.

76. Zhu J, Jiménez-Díaz J, Bean HD, et al. Robust detection of P. aeruginosa and S. aureus acute lung infections by secondary electrospray ionization-mass spectrometry (SESI-MS) breathprinting: from initial infection to clearance. J Breath Res 2013;7(3):37106.

77. van Oort PM, Brinkman P, Slingers G, et al. Exhaled breath metabolomics reveals a pathogen-specific response in a rat pneumonia model for two human pathogenic bacteria: a proof-of-concept study. Am J Physiol Cell Mol Physiol 2019; 316(5):L751–6.

78. Gisbert JP, Pajares JM. Review article: 13C-urea breath test in the diagnosis of Helicobacter pylori infection – a critical review. Aliment Pharmacol Ther 2004; 20(10):1001–17.

79. Maity A, Banik GD, Ghosh C, et al. Residual gas analyzer mass spectrometry for human breath analysis: a new tool for the non-invasive diagnosis of Helicobacter pylori infection. J Breath Res 2014;8(1):016005.

80. Gao J, Zou Y, Wang Y, et al. Breath analysis for noninvasively differentiating Acinetobacter baumannii ventilator-associated pneumonia from its respiratory tract colonization of ventilated patients. J Breath Res 2016;10(2):27102.

81. Zhu J, Bean HD, Wargo MJ, et al. Detecting bacterial lung infections: in vivo evaluation of in vitro volatile fingerprints. J Breath Res 2013;7(1):16003.

82. Hockstein NG, Thaler ER, Torigian D, et al. Diagnosis of pneumonia with an electronic nose: correlation of vapor signature with chest computed tomography scan findings. Laryngoscope 2004;114(10):1701–5.

83. Hockstein NG, Thaler ER, Lin Y, et al. Correlation of pneumonia score with electronic nose signature: a prospective study. Ann Otol Rhinol Laryngol 2005;114(7): 504–8.

84. Filipiak W, Beer R, Sponring A, et al. Breath analysis for in vivo detection of pathogens related to ventilator-associated pneumonia in intensive care patients: a prospective pilot study. J Breath Res 2015;9(1):016004.

85. Fowler SJ, Basanta-Sanchez M, Xu Y, et al. Surveillance for lower airway pathogens in mechanically ventilated patients by metabolomic analysis of exhaled breath: a case-control study. Thorax 2015;70(4):320–5.

86. van Oort P, de Bruin S, Weda H, et al. Exhaled breath metabolomics for the diagnosis of pneumonia in Intubated and mechanically-ventilated intensive care unit (ICU)-Patients. Int J Mol Sci 2017;18(2):449.

87. Schnabel R, Fijten R, Smolinska A, et al. Analysis of volatile organic compounds in exhaled breath to diagnose ventilator-associated pneumonia. Sci Rep 2015; 5(1):17179.

88. Andrews BT, Das P, Denzer W, et al. Breath testing for intra-abdominal infection: appendicitis, a preliminary study. J Breath Res 2020;15(1):16002.

89. Acharige MJT, Koshy S, Ismail N, et al. Breath-based diagnosis of fungal infections. J Breath Res 2018;12(2):027108.

90. Sethi S, Nanda R, Chakraborty T. Clinical application of volatile organic compound analysis for detecting infectious diseases. Clin Microbiol Rev 2013; 26(3):462–75.

91. Chambers ST, Syhre M, Murdoch DR, et al. Detection of 2-Pentylfuran in the breath of patients with Aspergillus fumigatus. Med Mycol 2009;47(5):468–76.

92. Koo S, Thomas HR, Daniels SD, et al. A breath fungal secondary metabolite signature to diagnose invasive aspergillosis. Clin Infect Dis 2014;59(12):1733–40.

93. de Heer K, van der Schee MP, Zwinderman K, et al. Electronic nose technology for detection of invasive pulmonary aspergillosis in prolonged chemotherapy-induced neutropenia: a proof-of-principle study. J Clin Microbiol 2013;51(5):1490–5.
94. de Heer K, Kok MGM, Fens N, et al. Detection of airway colonization by Aspergillus fumigatus by use of electronic nose technology in patients with cystic fibrosis. J Clin Microbiol 2016;54(3):569–75.
95. Hertel M, Schuette E, Kastner I, et al. Volatile organic compounds in the breath of oral candidiasis patients: a pilot study. Clin Oral Investig 2018;22(2):721–31.

Clinical Mass Spectrometry Approaches to Myeloma and Amyloidosis

David L. Murray, MD, PhD[a],*, Surendra Dasari, PhD[b]

KEYWORDS

- Clinical mass spectrometry • Multiple myeloma • Amyloidosis • Proteomics
- Plasma cell disorders • MALDI-TOF mass spectrometry

KEY POINTS

- Mass spectrometric methods for multiple myeloma and amyloidosis are expanding knowledge of these diseases.
- A combination of bottom-up and top-down mass spectrometry methods is currently being used in the routine care of patients.
- As these methods continue to improve over time, they are likely to become the standard method for patient care.

BACKGROUND

Plasma cells are terminally differentiated B cells that produce large quantities of immunoglobulin (also called antibody; **Fig. 1**), which serves as the body's defense against foreign invaders. A plasma cell clone is defined by the unique immunoglobulin produced by that clone. The uniqueness of the immunoglobulin stems from the complementary determining region (CDR), which is an aptly suited N-terminal sequence for binding with a foreign protein. Before maturing into a plasma cell, B cells undergo somatic rearrangement of both the heavy chain and light chain (LC) immunoglobulin genes, resulting in a variation in sequence from the germ line. Once the B cell encounters a foreign antigen, a process of maturation ensues with the end result of a plasma cell clone. Determining the repertoire of plasma cell clones within a particular individual could provide insight into the diversity of antigen exposure. Because plasma cells mostly reside in bone marrow, attempting to determine the CDR sequence diversity by DNA sequencing is very difficult because plasma cell sampling is, at best, incomplete.[1] Plasma cells self-amplify their CDR region by producing large amounts of

[a] Department of Laboratory Medicine and Pathology, Mayo Clinic, Rochester, MN, USA;
[b] Department of Health Sciences Research, Mayo Clinic, Rochester, MN, USA
* Corresponding author.
E-mail address: murray.david@mayo.edu

Clin Lab Med 41 (2021) 203–219
https://doi.org/10.1016/j.cll.2021.03.003
0272-2712/21/© 2021 Elsevier Inc. All rights reserved.

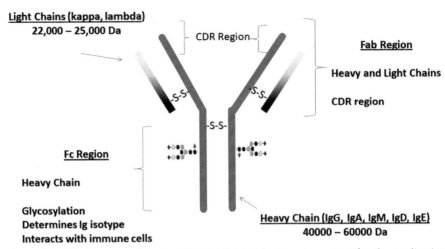

Fig. 1. Simplified immunoglobulin with highlighted features important for the application of mass spectrometry. CDR, complementary determining region; Ig, immunoglobulin.

immunoglobulins, which result in total serum immunoglobulin levels of 10 g/L. The unique sequence along with their high abundance in serum make immunoglobulins and plasma cell disorders (PCDs) an attractive target for current proteomics techniques.

PCDs are common in the general population. However, most patients with PCDs are asymptomatic and are in a category termed monoclonal gammopathy of undetermined significance (MGUS). Studies have shown that approximately 3% of individuals more than 50 years of age have MGUS.[2] Most of these individuals remain asymptomatic, with only 1% per year developing a PCD that requires treatment.[3] PCDs can be subdivided into frank malignancy (eg, multiple myeloma) and those that overproduce monoclonal immunoglobulins that are detrimental to the body (eg, primary systemic amyloidosis). In either case, treatment consists of eliminating the plasma cells responsible for the symptoms. Treatment can consist of traditional chemotherapy drugs, therapeutic monoclonal antibodies (t-mAbs), or autologous stem cell transplant.[4]

Key to making a diagnosis of a PCD is detection of the monoclonal immunoglobulin (also called M-protein or paraprotein) produced by the expanding plasma cell clone.[5] In the past, the detection of the M-protein has been accomplished using serum gel or capillary electrophoretic methods. These methods depend on the slight differences in the electrophoretic mobility of each immunoglobulin. Because immunoglobulins mainly interact with other proteins, the CDR region contains abundant basic Amino acids (AAs), which results in their migration close to the cathode. In normal individuals, the unique AA sequence of numerous immunoglobulins produces a distribution of charge and a broad migration pattern on the gel (**Fig. 2**A). When an overproduced monoclonal immunoglobulin is present, the result is a restricted band within this region (**Fig. 2**B) consistent with a PCD. Although electrophoretic methods have served well over the years, there is a need for improved sensitivity and specificity to keep pace with the modern myeloma treatment regimens, which are eradicating more and more of the aberrant plasma cells.[6]

Amyloidosis refers to a rare, complex, and ominous group of clinical syndromes that are caused by deposition of misfolded proteins in organs as β-pleated sheet fibrils. These fibrils cause cellular death and organ dysfunction as plaques accumulate within

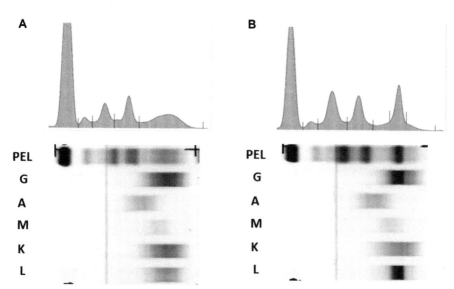

Fig. 2. Examples of a normal (*A*) and abnormal (*B*) serum protein electrophoresis (*top*) and immunofixation electrophoresis (*bottom*). Note the broad migration of the polyclonal immunoglobulin background in the normal (*A*) gamma region and the relatively restricted M-protein in the abnormal (*B*) patient. The immunofixation reveals an IgG kappa M-protein isotype.

the organs.[7] To date, 36 different proteins are recognized to have the potential to form these pathogenic fibrils.[8] The clinical manifestations of the amyloidosis are myriad,[9] subtle, and nonspecific, thus making the diagnosis difficult. Typically, patients whose symptoms are compatible with potential amyloidosis diagnosis undergo biopsy of involved organs.[10] The diagnosis of amyloidosis is confirmed by the identification of Congo red (CR)–positive amorphous protein deposits that have a characteristic apple-green birefringence under polarized light.[11] After establishing the diagnosis of amyloid, the primary amyloidogenic protein that seeded the deposit needs to be identified (also called typing) in order to prescribe a therapeutic course for the patient.[12] A wide variety of treatment courses are available, each of which is custom tailored for the amyloid type. For example, the most frequently seen amyloid type is systemic amyloid LC (AL) amyloidosis, which is caused by the deposition of immunoglobulin LCs produced by a malignant monotypic plasma cell population in the bone marrow. Hence, treatment of AL amyloidosis is directed at bone marrow, which includes chemotherapy and autologous bone marrow transplant.[13] The next most common systemic amyloid transthyretin amyloidosis is caused by deposition of wild-type monomeric unstable transthyretin (TTR) protein. Treatment of ATTR amyloidosis involves either a liver transplant or stabilizing the tetrameric structure of transthyretin using drugs.[14] Renal/liver transplants can be effective therapies for patients whose amyloid deposits contains mutated fibrinogen alpha (FIBA) protein,[15] which destabilizes the protein. In addition, some of the amyloid types, such as AA, which is caused by deposition of serum amyloid A protein (SAA), are managed via symptomatic treatment. Because of the wide-ranging options available for therapy, accurate typing of the amyloid deposit is essential for clinical management of the patient.

Historically, antibody-based methods such as immunohistochemistry, immunofluorescence, and immunoelectron microscopy have been used to type the amyloid deposit.[16,17] These methods suffer from a variety of technical limitations, all of which are traceable to their use of antibodies against 4 proteins (immunoglobulin kappa LC, immunoglobulin lambda LC, transthyretin, and serum amyloid A protein) that account for ~90% of the amyloid types seen in the clinic. The antibodies that are widely available for recognizing these proteins are not optimized for detecting the randomly truncated forms of proteins present in the amyloid deposit.[18–20] Further, the β-pleated sheet conformation of amyloid proteins also confers adhesive properties to the amyloid fibrils, resulting in nonspecific interaction between the antibodies and fibrils.[21] These factors combined together limit the sensitivity and specificity of detecting the proper amyloidogenic protein that is present in a deposit.

In this review, the role of traditional proteomics by mass spectrometry (MS) in diagnosing PCDs and subtyping amyloidosis is delineated as these techniques are currently being applied daily to the clinical care of patients with these disorders.

USE OF MASS SPECTROMETRY METHODS TO DETECT PLASMA CELL DISORDERS

The use of MS to analyze immunoglobulins emerged from efforts of the pharmaceutical industry to characterize t-mAbs.[22] This early work was mainly focused on characterizing pure t-mAbs with emphasis on determining chemical and structural features. In contrast, little work had been done on MS immunoglobulin characterization in human serum. The thought of detecting a single immunoglobulin clone in the midst of hundreds of thousands of similar immunoglobulin molecules is both a daunting and intriguing proposition. Several approaches have been devised and are summarized in **Fig. 3**.

The Clonotypic Peptide Approach

Building on the bottom-up proteomics work of Dekker and colleagues,[23] researchers have used M-protein immunoglobulin variable region/CDR tryptic (clonotypic) peptides to track and quantitate the presence of the M-protein in a cohort of treated patients with myeloma.[24–29] In all of the studies performed using this clonotypic peptide approach, disease-associated M-proteins were detected in the serum of treated patients with multiple myelomas that were not detected by traditional electrophoretic techniques. These results suggest that the clonotypic peptide method could be a viable method to test treated patients with myeloma for the presence of low-level disease or minimal residual disease (MRD). To date, a definite clinical study showing the impact of detecting low-level disease by the clonotypic peptide method in patients with myeloma is still pending.

Although the clonotypic method is analytically sensitive, the clonotypic approach has several drawbacks that make it difficult to implement in a routine clinical laboratory. First, a unique tryptic peptide from the CDR region of the M-protein must be identified and verified. In 1 study using de novo M-protein sequencing from patients with myeloma before their treatment, the identification of the clonotypic peptide was only feasible when the concentration of the M-protein was high enough (~8 g/L) to be readily recognized among the peptides from the polyclonal immunoglobulin background.[26] For some patients, a unique tryptic peptide may not be identified by de novo sequencing in spite of high concentrations of M-protein. Most of the clonotypic peptide studies in myeloma used CDR sequencing data from bone marrow biopsies to aid in identifying a unique peptide. Although these data add confidence in determining a unique CDR peptide, the data are not readily available for most patients with myeloma. The uniqueness of a single clonotypic peptide within an individual's polyclonal immunoglobulin repertoire is also a matter for verification, especially when the M-protein concentration decreases.

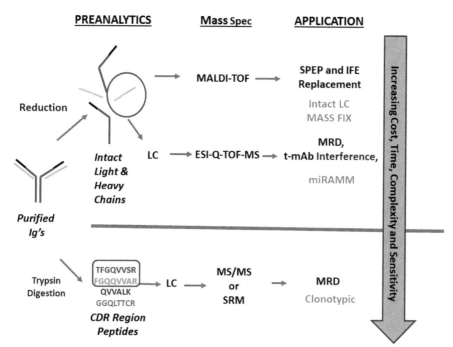

Fig. 3. An overview of the methods applied to characterize M-protein in serum. All methods start with immunoenrichment of the patient's immunoglobulins. Digestion with trypsin in the clonotypic method produces CDR-specific peptides that can be characterize by liquid chromatography tandem MS (MS/MS) and, once identified, can be followed by selective reaction monitoring (SRM). In the intact LC method, the mass distribution of the LCs can be used to detect M-proteins. Matrix-assisted laser desorption ionization (MALDI) time-of-flight (TOF) MS (MASS-FIX) has been adopted into laboratories in place of Serum Protein Electrophoresis (SPEP) and Immunofixation Electrophoresis (IFE). Higher-resolution liquid chromatography electrospray ionization (ESI) quadrupole (Q) TOF measurements (monoclonal immunoglobulin rapid accurate mass measurement) allows increased sensitivity and specificity for detecting low-level disease and distinguishing t-mAbs) from M-proteins. MRD, minimal residual disease.

A study on the polyclonal immunoglobulin CDR repertoire from 7 healthy individuals shown a total of 43,217 peptides in the polyclonal background.[30] Although this is a large number, only 17% of the peptides did not overlap with other patients. Combined with the total theoretically large number of possible of CDR rearrangements of 10^{23} and the similarity of the framework regions within the CDR, this fact lends credence to the caution in the use of a single CDR clonotypic peptide to detect low-level M-proteins.[31] Another limitation is the overall complexity of the clonotypic peptide method and its long preanalytical time making the clonotypic approach impractical as a screening method for M-proteins. This point is important given that the bulk of testing in any clinical laboratory is screening patients who are clinically suspected of having a PCD. At the time of this report, the authors are unaware of use of the clonotypic peptide method in the routine care of patients with myeloma.

The Intact Immunoglobulin Light Chain Middle-Down Approach

A second approach to detecting M-proteins that has been reported uses a middle-down or intact LC approach in which the immunoglobulin molecules are chemically reduced and the immunoglobulin LC mass distribution is queried for the presence of an M-protein[19] (see **Fig. 3**). In a sense, this method is more similar to electrophoretic detections because the M-protein presents as peak in the LC m/z mass distribution. Assessing the polyclonal background is important to making a diagnosis of a PCD and requires the immunoglobulin to be expressed more than the polyclonal background. Initial method development of the intact LC work focused on using immunoglobulin enrichment with chemical reduction followed by liquid chromatography electrospray ionization (ESI) quadrupole time-of-flight (TOF) MS (termed monoclonal immunoglobulin rapid accurate mass measurement [miRAMM] by the investigators).[32] Unlike electrophoresis, the m/z distribution of LCs results in 2 distinct broad distributions: 1 for kappa and 1 for lambda.[33] The separation into kappa and lambda mass distributions is one of the reasons for enhanced specificity of this approach. The miRAMM method was shown to work in both serum and urine.[34] Using miRAMM, the M-protein limit of detection could be improved compared with electrophoresis and the accurate molecular mass of the M-protein LC (measured within 1 Da) could be used as a personalized biomarker to track disease over years.[32] All these features show that the principle of using LC m/z distributions could enhance the ability to detect and monitor PCDs. However, the initial miRAMM approach still had some limitations hindering its ability to be used as a routine assay. The initial preanalytical step used a simple immunoenrichment resin (Melon Gel) that removes nonimmunoglobulin proteins from solution. However, specific immunoglobulin isotypes (in particular immunoglobulin A [IgA] isotypes) had poor recovery using Melon Gel. In addition, the use of intact mass of heavy chains (HCs) and LCs alone was insufficient to provide conclusive immunoglobulin isotype information. The determination of M-protein isotype is critical to help guide both the physicians and subsequent bone marrow studies on the patient. IgG-related and IgA-related PCDs are more typical of multiple myeloma, whereas IgM-related PCDs are typically related to lymphoplasmacytic lymphoma or Waldenström macroglobulinemia. The miRAMM method used chromatography to separate the immunoglobulins (~25 min/sample), hindering the number of patient samples that could be analyzed in a given day. In addition, because M-proteins can range in concentration from milligrams to grams per liter, carryover of an M-protein on the LC system was also a concern. To address these issues, the chromatography was eliminated and replaced with immunoenrichment, and the separate spots on a matrix-assisted laser desorption/ionization (MALDI) TOF MS plate lessened the concern for M-protein carryover.[35] The preanalytical method was modified to use immunoenrichments for both the immunoglobulin HC (ie, IgG, IgA, IgM) and the immunoglobulin LC (ie, kappa and lambda).[36,37] The immune enrichment was accomplished using agarose beads to which were coupled camelid-derived nanobodies. These nanobodies (derived from the camelid species) were preferred to other species because their molecular mass (approximately 13,500 Da) is outside the range of human immunoglobulin LCs (approximately 23,000–25,000 Da). This method enabled robust reduction and elution conditions where the unintended release of nanobodies from the agarose beads would not produce interference in the m/z spectra. Conventional antihuman immunoglobulin antibodies commonly used are raised in species (ie, mouse, horse, and goat) with overlapping immunoglobulin LC mass distributions.

The combination of immune-enrichment and MALDI-TOF MS methods (termed MASS-FIX and MASS-SCREEN at Mayo Clinic) have combined properties suited for the routine clinical laboratory. Analytical times are rapid (<1 minute per patient) and the assay can detect, quantitate, and isotype M-proteins. The analytical equipment (Bruker, Microflex MALDI-TOF) has also gained acceptance in the clinical laboratory for identification of bacteria and other pathogens. The overlapping of spectra from the separate immune enrichments allows the determination of the isotype (**Fig. 4**). The immunoenrichments also remove interfering proteins such as beta-migrating proteins and fibrinogen, which have hampered the detection of M-proteins by serum protein electrophoresis (SPEP).[38] Validation of a fully automated intact LC MALDI-TOF method to replace immunofixation has been described[39] and is currently used for patient care at the Mayo Clinic.

Before the intact LC MALDI-TOF MS method was adapted into clinical care, clinical studies comparing the method with traditional electrophoretic methods were performed. As a PCD screening method, serum MASS-FIX applied to 182 samples submitted for routine M-protein detection revealed that serum MASS-FIX had an analytical sensitivity equivalent to a panel of serum PEL, serum immunofixation, and Hevylite assay.[36] In a clinical sensitivity study, MASS-FIX in combination with serum free LC measurements (sFLC) or urine MASS-FIX had equal sensitivity to current International Myeloma Working Group (IMWG) recommended panels.[40] These clinical studies also showed a previously under-recognized feature of some M-proteins, LC N-linked glycosylation. These LC glycosylated M-proteins were first seen during screening and clinical studies as LCs with masses larger than expected. Follow-up studies using PNGase enzymes revealed that these LCs were N-linked glycosylated.[41] Patients with M-proteins having glycosylated LCs were found to be persistent through the long-term course of their disease[42] and their presence was shown to be a risk factor for AL amyloidosis, bleeding diathesis in myeloma,[43] and progression of MGUS to a PCD needing treatment.[44] In addition, IgM kappa M-proteins with kappa LC glycosylation have been implicated in a rare cause of hemolytic anemia, cold agglutinin disease.[45] The pathologic and clinical impacts of these modifications warrant further research.

In efforts to provide more sequence data on M-proteins, LC and heavy chain fragmentation patterns from tandem MS (MS/MS) methods were investigated using a high-resolution 21-T Fourier-transform ion cyclotron resonance instrument. Modified top-down and middle-down MS was able to provide broad sequence coverage, which enables extensive mapping and glycoprofiling of M-proteins.[46] In addition, LC

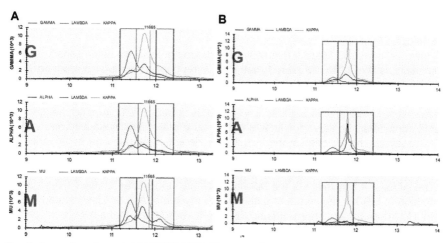

Fig. 4. Examples of overlaid MALDI-TOF MS spectra from 5 separate immune enrichments for IgG (*G, top, black*), IgA (*A, middle, black*), IgM (*M, bottom, black*) and kappa (*orange*) and lambda (*blue*) for a normal patient (*A*) and a patient with an IgA kappa M-protein (*B*).

sequencing information was also determined, which could provide enough detail to determine which monoclonal protein has a greater tendency to form amyloid.[47] These studies showed that such information on M-protein gene usage is feasible but the availability of such high accuracy mass spectrometers is very limited. Future work will most likely need to be performed on lower-cost instrumentation in order to bring this information to clinicians.

Another recent development in the treatment of multiple myeloma has been the use of t-mAbs to target and eliminate the malignant myeloma plasma cells.[48] These plasma cell targeting antibodies have proved to be highly effective and are quickly moving toward first-line therapy in myeloma.[49] Although these are benefiting patients, t-mAb treatments are interfering with the detection of the IgG kappa monoclonal M-proteins because the IgG kappa drugs can be difficult to distinguish from the IgG kappa M-proteins.[50–52] Although efforts to clear the interference on protein electrophoresis have been reported,[53] methods are currently limited to 1 drug, daratumumab, whereas several other t-mAbs are currently being used clinically. Several studies using MS have shown the usefulness of this method using both the clonotypic approach[27] and by using the intact LC approach.[54,55] The MS-based approaches are particular suited to being quickly adapted to new t-mAbs, because any new t-mAb can either be digested and a clonotypic peptide identified or chemically reduced and the LC mass measured.

In addition to electrophoretic methods for detecting M-proteins, the measurement of free kappa and lambda LCs is also broadly used in the detection and monitoring of patients with PCDs.[56] The IMWG has recommended a combination of electrophoresis and the free LC (FLC) measurements to be a part of the testing strategy to detect a PCD,[57] and the FLC test can aid in detecting patients with smoldering myeloma who need treatment.[58] The FLC assay has particular importance in detecting AL amyloidosis because an abnormal FLC ratio may be the only indicator of the disease.[59] Detection on monoclonal FLCs by this assay depends on observing a skewed kappa to lambda FLC ratio, which is an indirect indicator of an FLC M-protein. The intact LC method has been modified to detect monoclonal FLCs in a more direct measurement.[60] Compared with current electrophoretic identification of FLCs, immunoenrichment with FLC-specific reagents followed by the MALDI-TOF intact LC measurements improved the conformation of an abnormal FLC ratio significantly.[61] Use of MS identification of FLCs was also shown to be superior in detecting residual disease in AL amyloidosis.[62]

However, intact LC MALDI-TOF MS methods do not have the same sensitivity and resolution as the miRAMM-based methods. A retrospective study performed on a cohort of patients from Olmsted County, Minnesota, compared the ability of immunofixation electrophoresis, the intact MALDI-TOF, and miRAMM methodologies to detect early M-proteins in patients who later developed a PCD. Among the 226 patients considered negative for MGUS based on protein electrophoresis and serum FLC assay, a monoclonal protein could be detected at baseline in 24 patients (10.6%) by immunofixation, 113 patients (50%) by MADLI-TOF MS, and 149 patients (65.9%) by miRAMM MS.[63]

The increased sensitivity of the MS methods has spurred on studies investigating detection of MRD in the serum of patients with myeloma. As previously stated, treatments for myeloma are improving and there is renewed hope that a cure for myeloma may be possible, so attention to removing all traces of the disease becomes important. The current serum-based assays are not analytically sensitive enough for this purpose and some investigators have resorted to looking within the bone marrow aspirates for traces of disease.[64] Serum MRD studies using both the clonotypic method[26,29] and the intact LC method by MALDI-TOF[65] and the miRAMM method[66] have shown the potential of this approach to aid in detection of MRD. If successful, these methods could help reduce the need for costly and painful bone marrow biopsies.

USE OF MASS SPECTROMETRY FOR THE CHARACTERIZATION OF AMYLOID

Because of the criticality of accurate typing for clinical care and the unreliability of antibody-based methods, shotgun proteomics technology, which directly identifies proteins present in a sample, was explored for diagnostic purposes.[12,67–71] Vrana and colleagues[70] developed one of the early, clinically successful, methods for typing the amyloid using formalin-fixed paraffin-embedded (FFPE) tissue biopsies. This method, summarized in **Fig. 5**, started by isolating the CR-positive amyloid deposits from FFPE sections via laser microdissection for proteomics analysis. Proteins present in the microdissected FFPE material were extracted and denatured via heat and sonication. Extracted proteins were digested into peptides by an overnight incubation with porcine trypsin enzyme. Digested peptides were analyzed using a reverse-phase liquid chromatography coupled electrospray ionization enabled tandem MS (RPLC-ESI-MS/MS) method. Resulting tandem mass spectra were processed using a suite of sophisticated bioinformatics software to identify the peptides and proteins present in the amyloid deposit. The total number of MS/MS spectra that matched to each protein, a surrogate semiquantitative measure of a protein's abundance, present in the deposit was also tallied. The identification and quantification information of all proteins present in a patient's amyloid deposit was considered as the patient's personalized amyloid proteome.

A patient's amyloid proteome can be scrutinized to find the type deterministic amyloidogenic protein. **Fig. 6** shows amyloid proteomes obtained from 5 different patients,

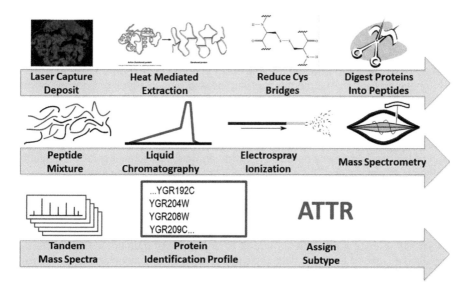

Fig. 5. Amyloid proteomic typing method for FFPE tissues. Tissue sections are CR stained and amyloid deposits are laser microdissected for shotgun proteomics analysis. An amyloid proteome is constructed from the data to identify the amyloidogenic protein present in the deposit and assign a subtype. Cys, cysteine.

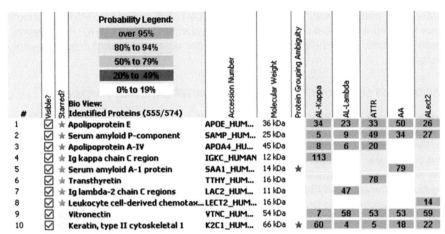

#	Visible?	Starred?	Bio View: Identified Proteins (555/574)	Accession Number	Molecular Weight	Protein Grouping Ambiguity	AL-Kappa	AL-Lambda	ATTR	AA	ALect2
1	☑	★	Apolipoprotein E	APOE_HUM...	36 kDa		34	23	33	50	26
2	☑	★	Serum amyloid P-component	SAMP_HUM...	25 kDa		5	9	49	34	27
3	☑	★	Apolipoprotein A-IV	APOA4_HU...	45 kDa		8	6	20		
4	☑	★	Ig kappa chain C region	IGKC_HUMAN	12 kDa		113				
5	☑	★	Serum amyloid A-1 protein	SAA1_HUM...	14 kDa	★				79	
6	☑	★	Transthyretin	TTHY_HUM...	16 kDa				78		
7	☑	★	Ig lambda-2 chain C regions	LAC2_HUM...	11 kDa			47			
8	☑	★	Leukocyte cell-derived chemotax...	LECT2_HUM...	16 kDa						14
9	☑		Vitronectin	VTNC_HUM...	54 kDa		7	58	53	53	59
10	☑		Keratin, type II cytoskeletal 1	K2C1_HUM...	66 kDa	★	60	4	5	18	22

Probability Legend:
over 95%
80% to 94%
50% to 79%
20% to 49%
0% to 19%

Fig. 6. Proteomic profiles of 5 different amyloid subtypes. All of the presented representative cases are FFPE biopsies. Kappa and lambda LC amyloidoses are presented separately here as AL-kappa and AL-lambda, respectively. Numbers in the green boxes indicate total number of MS/MS spectra matching a protein. APOE, SAP, and APOA4 are generic amyloid markers.

each with a distinct amyloid type. The universal amyloid chaperone proteins (apolipoprotein A4, apolipoprotein E, and serum amyloid P component) were detected in all amyloid types. These 3 proteins are considered to be a universal molecular signature for amyloid tissue. In contrast, type deterministic proteins were detected only in patients' deposits of corresponding subtype. For example, immunoglobulin kappa LC protein was detected only in deposits of AL-kappa subtype, immunoglobulin lambda LC protein was detected only in deposits of AL-lambda subtype, transthyretin protein was detected only in deposits of ATTR subtype, serum amyloid A-1 protein was detected only in deposits of AA subtype, and leukocyte cell–derived chemotaxin-2 protein was detected only in deposits of ALECT2 subtype. This specificity of subtype deterministic proteins, combined with the ability of shotgun proteomics to detect them in an unbiased fashion, makes the platform ideal for amyloid typing. Because of the success of the FFPE-based amyloid proteomic typing, methods were also developed to perform typing using subcutaneous fat aspirate specimens.[67,71]

Another advantage of MS-based methods for amyloid typing is their ability to detect pathogenic mutations present in the amyloidogenic proteins.[72] This ability signals the origin of the amyloidosis as hereditary, triggering genetic counseling for the patients and their family members. There are hundreds of pathogenic mutations that are known to occur in amyloidogenic proteins,[73] and approximately 19% of the non-AL amyloidosis subtypes can have a pathogenic mutation in the amyloidogenic proteins, signaling hereditary amyloidosis. Antibody-based methods cannot detect the presence of these mutations in patient specimens. In contrast, the amyloid MS data contain all the information that is needed to detect these mutations. Researchers[72] have used advanced bioinformatics tools and protein sequence databases to interrogate the MS data for presence of the known pathogenic mutations in amyloidogenic proteins. These methods showed very high sensitivity (>90%) and specificity (100%). Bioinformatics methods were also developed to detect novel, pathogenic, single-amino-acid substitutions in amyloidogenic proteins when the index of suspicion is high for hereditary amyloidosis and no known pathogenic mutations were detected in the patient's specimen.[72,74–78] These mutation detection methods do have limitations because they cannot detect truncations, novel frame shifts, isobaric mutations, and mutations that are in peptides not accessible by protein digestion enzymes. Despite these shortcomings, the ability of proteomics-based methods to find most known pathogenic mutations in a large fraction of the patients is valuable for properly diagnosing hereditary amyloidosis subtypes and prescribing a proper course of action for the patients and their families.

AL amyloidosis, the most commonly occurring amyloidosis subtype, is characterized by production of a pathogenic LC that is deposited in end organs, such as heart and kidney, causing organ damage (as described earlier). It has been hypothesized that the variable region of the LC is a key determinant of its pathogenicity and target end organ (organotropism). There are ~70 different LC variable (LCV) region genes, from which 1 gene is selected and hypermutated to encode for the LC of an immunoglobulin clone. Before the development of MS for amyloid typing, there were no methods that could detect the LCV gene of the LC present in the deposit. Researchers[47] have developed methods that can analyze amyloid MS data and infer the LCV gene encoding the pathogenic LC. These methods use generic sequence templates corresponding with LCV genes and do not require an a priori analysis of the patient's bone marrow plasma cells via next-generation sequencing to determine the LCV repertoire. This method led to the deployment of LCV gene detection workflow for AL patients in routine clinical care and the LCV of pathogenic LC can be inferred in ~80% of the AL patients, with 100% specificity.[47] Researchers used this workflow to study LCV gene usage patterns of AL clones in a large patient population and showed that certain LCV genes are more predisposed toward producing a pathogenic clone, and AL clones made from specific LCV genes can target specific organs.[79] In addition, the clonality (monoclonal vs polyclonal) of LC present in a deposit can be determined. When a single LCV gene is detected in an AL deposit, it implies that the pathogenic LC is derived from a clonal B-cell/plasma cell process, which is the case for primary systemic AL amyloidosis characterized by a bone marrow–based clonal plasma cell proliferation. In contrast, if multiple LCV genes are detected in an AL deposit, it implies the process is polyclonal (eg, laryngotracheal amyloidosis) and explains the indolent/localized nature of that disease.[80,81] Distinguishing between a systemic AL versus a localized AL is important because the treatments and outcomes for them are vastly different. This type of precise analysis is not feasible when using antibody-based methods and it clearly shows the superiority of shotgun proteomics–based amyloid typing in delivering tailored patient care for AL patients.

The shotgun proteomics–based method, because it is unbiased, is ideally suited for finding novel amyloidosis subtypes. Over the years, researchers have used the method to find novel amyloidosis subtypes caused by genes that were hitherto not known to have amyloidogenic potential. Examples include LECT2,[82,83] APOC2,[74,76] APOA4,[84] APOC3,[78] APOA2,[85] EFEMP1,[86] and pharmaceutical insulin.[8] Discovering new amyloid subtypes is significantly difficult when using antibody-based typing methods because it requires a priori knowledge of the target gene and availability of a working antibody for precisely detecting its protein product in an amyloid deposit.

Technological advantages of shotgun proteomics and associated bioinformatics have made MS ideally suited for typing amyloid fibrils. This method can be performed using FFPE or subcutaneous fat aspirate specimens and it has marked advantages compared with antibody-based methods. It detects all known amyloid types in a single assay and can be used to detect pathogenic mutations and LCV genes of AL clones, neither of which is possible to accomplish via antibody-based methods. As a testament to its robustness and relevance to patient care, shotgun proteomics–based amyloid typing is now accepted worldwide as standard of care for typing amyloid fibrils.[10,12,67–69]

SUMMARY

The detection of M-proteins and subtyping of amyloid deposits using MS are good examples of how MS has gone beyond the well-established LC-MS identification of drugs and vitamin D in the clinical laboratory. In these applications, several key aspects of the benefit of MS were used to advance understanding of the diseases. For M-proteins, the increased resolution and sensitivity of modern TOFs and Orbitrap instruments have allowed the detection of single immunoglobulin clones within a diverse repertoire of polyclonal antibodies. The ability to further characterize the tertiary structure of M-proteins has shed light on post translation modification, such as LC glycosylation, which were likely always present in patients with myeloma but went undetected by previous methods. These findings are broadening the understanding of PCDs. The ability to sample deeper into the proteome in a less blinded manner than immunohistochemistry has also shed light onto new proteins that are capable of forming amyloid, broadening knowledge of these diseases. Although the march of proteomics into the clinical laboratory has had its ups and downs, the methods in this article are translating into real patient care benefits and show that MS can be made practical and provide benefits for patient care.

CLINICS CARE POINTS

- Patients with multiple myeloma can be followed by newer mass spectrometric methods.
- Mass Spectrometry provides improved specificity in finding M-proteins.
- Mass Spectrometry provides improved specificity in discrimination therapeutic monoclonal drugs that other techniques.
- Mass Spectrometry has improved accuracy for typing amyloid plaques.
- Mass Spectrometry characterization of amyloid deposits has lead to discovery of new types of amyloid.

FUNDING

Work performed was funded by the Mayo Clinic.

DISCLOSURE

The authors have intellectual property rights on the use of MS in monoclonal gammopathies licensed to The Binding Site.

REFERENCES

1. Jiang N, Weinstein JA, Penland L, et al. Determinism and stochasticity during maturation of the zebrafish antibody repertoire. Proc Natl Acad Sci U S A 2011;108(13):5348–53.
2. Kyle RA, Therneau TM, Rajkumar SV, et al. Prevalence of monoclonal gammopathy of undetermined significance. N Engl J Med 2006;354(13):1362–9.

3. Kyle RA, Therneau TM, Rajkumar SV, et al. A long-term study of prognosis in monoclonal gammopathy of undetermined significance. N Engl J Med 2002; 346(8):564–9.

4. Moreau P, Touzeau C, Vij R, et al. Newly diagnosed myeloma in 2020. Am Soc Clin Oncol Educ Book 2020;40:1–15.

5. Willrich MAV, Murray DL, Kyle RA. Laboratory testing for monoclonal gammopathies: focus on monoclonal gammopathy of undetermined significance and smoldering multiple myeloma. Clin Biochem 2018;51:38–47.

6. Zajec M, Langerhorst P, VanDuijn MM, et al. Mass spectrometry for identification, monitoring, and minimal residual disease detection of M-proteins. Clin Chem 2020;66(3):421–33.

7. Merlini G, Bellotti V. Molecular mechanisms of amyloidosis. N Engl J Med 2003; 349(6):583–96.

8. Benson MD, Buxbaum JN, Eisenberg DS, et al. Amyloid nomenclature 2018: recommendations by the International Society of Amyloidosis (ISA) nomenclature committee. Amyloid 2018;25(4):215–9.

9. Palladini G, Merlini G. Systemic amyloidoses: what an internist should know. Eur J Intern Med 2013;24(8):729–39.

10. Picken MM. Modern approaches to the treatment of amyloidosis: the critical importance of early detection in surgical pathology. Adv Anat Pathol 2013; 20(6):424–39.

11. Mollee P, Renaut P, Gottlieb D, et al. How to diagnose amyloidosis. Intern Med J 2014;44(1):7–17.

12. Mollee P, Boros S, Loo D, et al. Implementation and evaluation of amyloidosis subtyping by laser-capture microdissection and tandem mass spectrometry. Clin Proteomics 2016;13:30.

13. Gertz MA. Immunoglobulin light chain amyloidosis diagnosis and treatment algorithm 2018. Blood Cancer J 2018;8(5):44.

14. Gertz MA, Mauermann ML, Grogan M, et al. Advances in the treatment of hereditary transthyretin amyloidosis: a review. Brain Behav 2019;9(9):e01371.

15. Gillmore JD, Lachmann HJ, Rowczenio D, et al. Diagnosis, pathogenesis, treatment, and prognosis of hereditary fibrinogen A alpha-chain amyloidosis. J Am Soc Nephrol 2009;20(2):444–51.

16. Solomon A, Murphy CL, Westermark P. Unreliability of immunohistochemistry for typing amyloid deposits. Arch Pathol Lab Med 2008;132(1):14 [author reply 14-5].

17. Satoskar AA, Burdge K, Cowden DJ, et al. Typing of amyloidosis in renal biopsies: diagnostic pitfalls. Arch Pathol Lab Med 2007;131(6):917–22.

18. Bergstrom J, Gustavsson A, Hellman U, et al. Amyloid deposits in transthyretin-derived amyloidosis: cleaved transthyretin is associated with distinct amyloid morphology. J Pathol 2005;206(2):224–32.

19. Gustafsson S, Ihse E, Henein MY, et al. Amyloid fibril composition as a predictor of development of cardiomyopathy after liver transplantation for hereditary transthyretin amyloidosis. Transplantation 2012;93(10):1017–23.

20. Mangione PP, Porcari R, Gillmore JD, et al. Proteolytic cleavage of Ser52Pro variant transthyretin triggers its amyloid fibrillogenesis. Proc Natl Acad Sci U S A 2014;111(4):1539–44.

21. Picken MM, Herrera GA. The burden of "sticky" amyloid: typing challenges. Arch Pathol Lab Med 2007;131(6):850–1.

22. Murray D, Barnidge D. Characterization of immunoglobulin by mass spectrometry with applications for the clinical laboratory. Crit Rev Clin Lab Sci 2013; 50(4–5):91–102.
23. Dekker LJM, Zeneyedpour L, Brouwer E, et al. An antibody-based biomarker discovery method by mass spectrometry sequencing of complementarity determining regions. Anal Bioanal Chem 2010;399(3):1081–91.
24. Barnidge DR, Tschumper RC, Theis JD, et al. Monitoring M-proteins in patients with multiple myeloma using heavy-chain variable region clonotypic peptides and LC-MS/MS. J Proteome Res 2014 4;13(4):1905-10.
25. Remily-Wood ER, Benson K, Baz RC, et al. Quantification of peptides from immunoglobulin constant and variable regions by LC-MRM MS for assessment of multiple myeloma patients. Proteomics Clin Appl 2014;8(9–10):783–95.
26. Bergen HR 3rd, Dasari S, Dispenzieri A, et al. Clonotypic light chain peptides identified for monitoring minimal residual disease in multiple myeloma without bone marrow aspiration. Clin Chem 2016;62(1):243–51.
27. Zajec M, Jacobs JFM, Groenen P, et al. Development of a targeted mass-spectrometry serum assay to quantify M-protein in the presence of therapeutic monoclonal antibodies. J Proteome Res 2018;17(3):1326–33.
28. Zajec M, Jacobs JFM, de Kat Angelino CM, et al. Integrating serum protein electrophoresis with mass spectrometry, A new workflow for M-protein detection and quantification. J Proteome Res 2020 Jul 2;19(7):2845-53.
29. Martins CO, Huet S, Yi SS, et al. Mass spectrometry-based method targeting Ig variable regions for assessment of minimal residual disease in multiple myeloma. J Mol Diagn 2020;22(7):901–11.
30. de Costa D, Broodman I, Vanduijn MM, et al. Sequencing and quantifying IgG fragments and antigen-binding regions by mass spectrometry. J Proteome Res 2010;9(6):2937–45.
31. Lefranc MP. Immunoglobulin and T Cell receptor genes: IMGT((R)) and the birth and rise of immunoinformatics. Front Immunol 2014;5:22.
32. Barnidge DR, Dasari S, Botz CM, et al. Using mass spectrometry to monitor monoclonal immunoglobulins in patients with a monoclonal gammopathy. J Proteome Res 2014 Mar 7;13(3):1419-27.
33. Barnidge DR, Dasari S, Ramirez-Alvarado M, et al. Phenotyping polyclonal kappa and lambda light chain molecular mass distributions in patient serum using mass spectrometry. J Proteome Res 2014;13(11):5198–205.
34. Botz CM, Barnidge DR, Murray DL, et al. Detecting monoclonal light chains in urine: microLC-ESI-Q-TOF mass spectrometry compared to immunofixation electrophoresis. Br J Haematol 2014;167(3):437–8.
35. Barnidge DR, Griffin TJ, Murray DL. Using matrix-assisted laser desorption/ionization time-of-flight mass spectrometry to detect monoclonal immunoglobulin light chains in serum and urine. Rapid Commun Mass Spectrom 2015;29:1–4.
36. Mills JR, Kohlhagen MC, Dasari S, et al. Comprehensive assessment of M-proteins using nanobody enrichment coupled to MALDI-TOF mass spectrometry. Clin Chem 2016;62(10):1334–44.
37. Kohlhagen MC, Barnidge DR, Mills JR, et al. Screening method for M-proteins in serum using nanobody enrichment coupled to MALDI-TOF mass spectrometry. Clin Chem 2016;62(10):1345–52.
38. McCudden CR, Jacobs JFM, Keren D, et al. Recognition and management of common, rare, and novel serum protein electrophoresis and immunofixation interferences. Clin Biochem 2018;51:72–9.

39. Kohlhagen M, Dasari S, Willrich M, et al. Automation and validation of a MALDI-TOF MS (Mass-Fix) replacement of immunofixation electrophoresis in the clinical lab. Clin Chem Lab Med 2020.
40. Milani P, Murray DL, Barnidge DR, et al. The utility of MASS-FIX to detect and monitor monoclonal proteins in the clinic. Am J Hematol 2017;92(8):772–9.
41. Kumar S, Murray D, Dasari S, et al. Assay to rapidly screen for immunoglobulin light chain glycosylation: a potential path to earlier AL diagnosis for a subset of patients. Leukemia 2019;33(1):254–7.
42. Kourelis T, Murray DL, Dasari S, et al. MASS-FIX may allow identification of patients at risk for light chain amyloidosis before the onset of symptoms. Am J Hematol 2018;93(11):E368–70.
43. Saadalla A, Seheult J, Ladwig PM, et al. Sialic acid bearing paraproteins are implicated in Heparin-like Coagulopathy in myeloma patients. Blood 2020 Oct 22;136(17):1988-92.
44. Dispenzieri A, Larson DR, Rajkumar SV, et al. N-glycosylation of monoclonal light chains on routine MASS-FIX testing is a risk factor for MGUS progression. Leukemia 2020 Oct;34(10):2749-53.
45. Sidana S, Murray DL, Dasari S, et al. Glycosylation of immunoglobulin light chains is highly prevalent in cold agglutinin disease. Am J Hematol 2020 Sep;95(9):E222-E225. http://doi.org/10.1002/ajh.25843. Epub 2020 Jun 12.
46. He L, Anderson LC, Barnidge DR, et al. Analysis of monoclonal antibodies in human serum as a model for clinical monoclonal gammopathy by use of 21 tesla FT-ICR top-down and middle-down MS/MS. J Am Soc Mass Spectrom 2017;28(5):827–38.
47. Dasari S, Theis JD, Vrana JA, et al. Proteomic detection of immunoglobulin light chain variable region peptides from amyloidosis patient biopsies. J Proteome Res 2015;14(4):1957–67.
48. Touzeau C, Moreau P, Dumontet C. Monoclonal antibody therapy in multiple myeloma. Leukemia 2017;31(5):1039–47.
49. Ludwig H. Daratumumab: a game changer in myeloma therapy. Lancet Haematol 2020;7(6):e426–7.
50. Mills JR, Murray DL. Identification of friend or foe: the laboratory Challenge of differentiating M-proteins from monoclonal antibody therapies. J Appl Lab Med 2017;1(4):421–31.
51. Willrich MA, Ladwig PM, Andreguetto BD, et al. Monoclonal antibody therapeutics as potential interferences on protein electrophoresis and immunofixation. Clin Chem Lab Med 2016;54(6):1085–93.
52. Murata K, McCash SI, Carroll B, et al. Treatment of multiple myeloma with monoclonal antibodies and the dilemma of false positive M-spikes in peripheral blood. Clin Biochem 2018 Jan;51:66-71.
53. McCudden C, Axel AE, Slaets D, et al. Monitoring multiple myeloma patients treated with daratumumab: teasing out monoclonal antibody interference. Clin Chem Lab Med 2016;54(6):1095–104.
54. Mills JR, Kohlhagen MC, Willrich MAV, et al. A universal solution for eliminating false positives in myeloma due to therapeutic monoclonal antibody interference. Blood 2018;132(6):670–2.
55. Moore LM, Cho S, Thoren KL. MALDI-TOF mass spectrometry distinguishes daratumumab from M-proteins. Clin Chim Acta 2019;492:91–4.
56. Bradwell AR, Carr-Smith HD, Mead GP, et al. Highly sensitive, automated immunoassay for immunoglobulin free light chains in serum and urine. Clin Chem 2001;47(4):673–80.

57. Dimopoulos M, Kyle R, Fermand JP, et al. Consensus recommendations for standard investigative workup: report of the international myeloma Workshop Consensus panel 3. Blood 2011;117(18):4701–5.

58. Rajkumar SV, Dimopoulos MA, Palumbo A, et al. International Myeloma Working Group updated criteria for the diagnosis of multiple myeloma. Lancet Oncol 2014;15(12):e538–48.

59. Katzmann JA, Kyle RA, Benson J, et al. Screening panels for detection of monoclonal gammopathies. Clin Chem 2009;55(8):1517–22.

60. Barnidge DR, Dispenzieri A, Merlini G, et al. Monitoring free light chains in serum using mass spectrometry. Clin Chem Lab Med 2016;54(6):1073–83.

61. Sepiashvili L, Kohlhagen MC, Snyder MR, et al. Direct detection of monoclonal free light chains in serum by use of immunoenrichment-coupled MALDI-TOF mass spectrometry. Clin Chem 2019;65(8):1015–22.

62. Dispenzieri A, Arendt B, Dasari S, et al. Blood mass spectrometry detects residual disease better than standard techniques in light-chain amyloidosis. Blood Cancer J 2020;10(2):20.

63. Murray D, Kumar SK, Kyle RA, et al. Detection and prevalence of monoclonal gammopathy of undetermined significance: a study utilizing mass spectrometry-based monoclonal immunoglobulin rapid accurate mass measurement. Blood Cancer J 2019;9(12):102.

64. Kostopoulos IV, Ntanasis-Stathopoulos I, Gavriatopoulou M, et al. Minimal residual disease in multiple myeloma: current landscape and future applications with immunotherapeutic approaches. Front Oncol 2020;10:860.

65. Eveillard M, Rustad E, Roshal M, et al. Comparison of MALDI-TOF mass spectrometry analysis of peripheral blood and bone marrow-based flow cytometry for tracking measurable residual disease in patients with multiple myeloma. Br J Haematol 2020;189(5):904–7.

66. Mills JR, Barnidge DR, Dispenzieri A, et al. High sensitivity blood-based M-protein detection in sCR patients with multiple myeloma. Blood Cancer J 2017; 7(8):e590.

67. Brambilla F, Lavatelli F, Di Silvestre D, et al. Reliable typing of systemic amyloidoses through proteomic analysis of subcutaneous adipose tissue. Blood 2012; 119(8):1844–7.

68. Gilbertson JA, Theis JD, Vrana JA, et al. A comparison of immunohistochemistry and mass spectrometry for determining the amyloid fibril protein from formalin-fixed biopsy tissue. J Clin Pathol 2015;68(4):314–7.

69. Murphy CL, Wang S, Williams T, et al. Characterization of systemic amyloid deposits by mass spectrometry. Methods Enzymol 2006;412:48–62.

70. Vrana JA, Gamez JD, Madden BJ, et al. Classification of amyloidosis by laser microdissection and mass spectrometry-based proteomic analysis in clinical biopsy specimens. Blood 2009;114(24):4957–9.

71. Vrana JA, Theis JD, Dasari S, et al. Clinical diagnosis and typing of systemic amyloidosis in subcutaneous fat aspirates by mass spectrometry-based proteomics. Haematologica 2014;99(7):1239–47.

72. Dasari S, Theis JD, Vrana JA, et al. Clinical proteome informatics workbench detects pathogenic mutations in hereditary amyloidoses. J Proteome Res 2014; 13(5):2352–8.

73. Rowczenio DM, Noor I, Gillmore JD, et al. Online registry for mutations in hereditary amyloidosis including nomenclature recommendations. Hum Mutat 2014; 35(9):E2403–12.

74. Nasr SH, Dasari S, Hasadsri L, et al. Novel type of renal amyloidosis derived from apolipoprotein-CII. J Am Soc Nephrol 2017;28(2):439–45.

75. Nasr SH, Dasari S, Mills JR, et al. Hereditary lysozyme amyloidosis variant p.Leu102Ser Associates with unique Phenotype. J Am Soc Nephrol 2017;28(2): 431–8.

76. Sethi S, Dasari S, Plaisier E, et al. Apolipoprotein CII amyloidosis associated with p.Lys41Thr mutation. Kidney Int Rep 2018;3(5):1193–201.

77. Sridharan M, Highsmith WE, Kurtin PJ, et al. A patient with hereditary ATTR and a novel AGel p.Ala578Pro amyloidosis. Mayo Clin Proc 2018;93(11):1678–82.

78. Valleix S, Verona G, Jourde-Chiche N, et al. D25V apolipoprotein C-III variant causes dominant hereditary systemic amyloidosis and confers cardiovascular protective lipoprotein profile. Nat Commun 2016;7:10353.

79. Kourelis TV, Dasari S, Theis JD, et al. Clarifying immunoglobulin gene usage in systemic and localized immunoglobulin light-chain amyloidosis by mass spectrometry. Blood 2017;129(3):299–306.

80. Grogg KL, Aubry MC, Vrana JA, et al. Nodular pulmonary amyloidosis is characterized by localized immunoglobulin deposition and is frequently associated with an indolent B-cell lymphoproliferative disorder. Am J Surg Pathol 2013;37(3): 406–12.

81. Ravindran A, Grogg KL, Domaas DA, et al. Polyclonal localized light chain amyloidosis-A distinct Entity? Clin Lymphoma Myeloma Leuk 2016;16(10): 588–92.

82. Benson MD, James S, Scott K, et al. Leukocyte chemotactic factor 2: a novel renal amyloid protein. Kidney Int 2008;74(2):218–22.

83. Mereuta OM, Theis JD, Vrana JA, et al. Leukocyte cell-derived chemotaxin 2 (LECT2)-associated amyloidosis is a frequent cause of hepatic amyloidosis in the United States. Blood 2014;123(10):1479–82.

84. Bois MC, Dasari S, Mills JR, et al. Apolipoprotein A-IV-associated Cardiac amyloidosis. J Am Coll Cardiol 2017;69(17):2248–9.

85. Prokaeva T, Akar H, Spencer B, et al. Hereditary renal amyloidosis associated with a novel apolipoprotein A-II variant. Kidney Int Rep 2017;2(6):1223–32.

86. Tasaki M, Ueda M, Hoshii Y, et al. A novel age-related venous amyloidosis derived from EGF-containing fibulin-like extracellular matrix protein 1. J Pathol 2019;247(4):444–55.

Breaking Through the Barrier

Regulatory Considerations Relevant to Ambient Mass Spectrometry at the Bedside

Michael Woolman, BSc[a,b], Lauren Katz, MSc[a,b],
Alessandra Tata, PhD[c], Sankha S. Basu, MD, PhD[d],
Arash Zarrine-Afsar, PhD[a,b,e,f],*

KEYWORDS

- Ambient mass spectrometry • Regulatory considerations
- Untargeted mass spectrometry analysis • Mass spectrometry in the clinic

KEY POINTS

- Regulatory recommendations for ambient mass spectrometry methods to be used at the bedside.
- Safety considerations for use of ambient MS methods in clinical settings.
- Harmonized validation workflow for evaluation of untargeted mass spectrometry methods.

AMBIENT MASS SPECTROMETRY IN CLINICAL APPLICATIONS; STATE OF THE ART

Ambient ionization mass spectrometry (MS) refers to techniques in which samples are analyzed under ambient conditions (ie, atmospheric pressure, room temperature) with little or no sample preparation, allowing high-throughput analysis of samples under native conditions. In the context of future clinical applications, ambient MS methods

[a] Techna Institute for the Advancement of Technology for Health, University Health Network, 100 College Street, Toronto, Ontario M5G 1P5, Canada; [b] Department of Medical Biophysics, University of Toronto, 101 College Street, Toronto, Ontario M5G 1L7, Canada; [c] Laboratorio di Chimica Sperimentale, Istituto Zooprofilattico delle Venezie, Viale Fiume 78, 36100 Vicenza, Italy; [d] Department of Pathology, Brigham and Women's Hospital, Harvard Medical School, Boston, MA 02115, USA; [e] Department of Surgery, University of Toronto, 149 College Street, Toronto, Ontario M5T 1P5, Canada; [f] Keenan Research Center for Biomedical Science & the Li Ka Shing Knowledge Institute, St. Michael's Hospital, 30 Bond Street, Toronto, Ontario M5B 1W8, Canada
* Corresponding author: Prof. Arash Zarrine-Afsar, 101 College Street, Room 7-207, MaRS Building, Princess Margaret Cancer Research Tower, 7th floor (STTARR), Toronto, ON M5G 1L7.
E-mail address: arash.zarrine.afsar@utoronto.ca

Clin Lab Med 41 (2021) 221–246
https://doi.org/10.1016/j.cll.2021.03.004
0272-2712/21/© 2021 Elsevier Inc. All rights reserved.

allow direct access to biological tissues without lengthy sample preparation.[1] A typical ambient MS analysis workflow involves untargeted interrogation of tissue small molecule content and comparison (via multivariate statistical analysis) of a query m/z profile to a previously established and validated (via anatomic or molecular pathology) library of m/z profiles for various tissue disorders. Capitalizing on the close relationship between cancer formation and changes in lipid metabolism,[2] analysis of the lipidome by ambient MS methods to predict disorder has constituted the bulk of those reported in the literature.[1,3–16] Although most reported applications use untargeted analysis and changes in the entire mass range profile to highlight disorder, certain targeted applications using oncometabolites have been reported as well.[8–10,17,18] Although ambient MS methods allow unprecedented access to rapid (within few seconds), on-the-spot information regarding tissue disorder with high (>98%) specificity in certain cases,[1,15,16] the added value of using this real-time information in clinical decision making is not yet validated against patient outcomes. However, ambient MS methods in diagnostics have been used in 2 broad categories of point sampling and imaging modes. Point sampling approaches often use a handheld desorption source (or probe) affixed to a mass spectrometer for processing desorbed bulk tissue (either in or ex vivo). In contrast, the imaging mode commonly involves using an x-y translation stage to raster the desorption probe over an ex vivo tissue piece (often in the form of a flat slice) to generate a two-dimensional, spatially resolved image of the tissue molecular content. Although point sampling methods may be combined with three-dimensional tracking technologies to obtain spatially resolved information from in vivo tissue sampled in situ,[19] this hybrid mode has just been reported and is not widely used or evaluated.

Although a large number of different ambient MS sources exist,[15,16,20] including aerosols produced by surgical aspirators,[21] most are based on either liquid extraction (eg, desorption electrospray ionization,[22] MasSpec Pen[14]) or direct coupling between laser ablation (eg, picosecond infrared laser [PIRL] MS,[7] SpiderMass[12]) and MS or that of electrocautery[11] or rapid evaporative ionization MS (REIMS).[23,24] Ambient MS sources that use strong solvents or require significant electric fields at the probe tip to facilitate desorption or ionization have limitations that preclude them from immediate use in vivo without further modifications. However, recent developments of water-based extraction methods, such as the MasSpec Pen,[14] have revived interest in revisiting the role of solvent in ambient MS methods. A detailed description of ambient MS sources and technological advancements that have given rise to their developments are available elsewhere[1,15,16,25] and are not discussed further herein.

Ambient MS has experienced a significant horizontal growth throughout the recent decade, with no single source or method having broken through the regulatory barrier for approved clinical use. This article describes challenges associated with standardizing a validation workflow, and reviews concerns that must be addressed to facilitate approval, using 3 major clinical use case scenarios selected from the literature: assessment of biopsy adequacy, and clinical decision making using in vivo and ex vivo sampling.[1] The regulatory considerations that each envisioned scenario may require are highlighted to also draw attention to the potential of ambient MS to form the core technology of future clinical devices. Parallels are drawn from recent approvals of nonambient MS methods for microbial identification[26,27] as a potential alternative avenue to the laboratory-developed test (LDT) strategies that have formed the core of many targeted MS-based assays.[28] Guidelines from the US Pharmacopeia[29] (USP Pharmacopeial Convention, 2016, pp. 2053–2067) for validation of untargeted methods in food quality control (QC) are also discussed because they represent a close match with where ambient MS currently stands with respect to the need for harmonized validation protocols. This article further provides suggestions and additional considerations that may be relevant in systematic evaluation of ambient MS methods in clinical settings, especially for surgical guidance, which is reviewed elsewhere.[1]

REGULATORY CONSIDERATIONS IN MASS SPECTROMETRY–BASED ASSAYS: STATE OF THE ART

Before discussing specific regulatory considerations for ambient MS, it is worth briefly considering the current landscape of clinical MS and the regulatory and validation requirements needed for their implementation and widespread deployment. Note that both LDT and US Food and Drug Administration (FDA) approved tests have been proved to be viable avenues for MS-based assay compliance. There are 3 widely available and regulated clinical applications of MS. The first involves use of liquid chromatography tandem MS (LC-MS/MS) for analysis of drugs or endogenous metabolites, such as vitamin D[30], in body fluids such as serum or urine. The second is the use of gas chromatography (GC) MS[31] for newborn screening of inborn errors of metabolism. The third is a matrix-assisted laser desorption ionization (MALDI) time-of-flight (TOF) MS for microbial identification.[26,27] There are other clinical MS applications, but they are either in preclinical stages or have only been deployed at a limited number of centers.

The first 2 approaches (LC-MS/MS and GC-MS), represent targeted analyses in which a specific analyte or (in the case of multiplexed methods) a set of analytes is being quantified within a specified biological matrix. This analysis is most commonly performed using triple quadrupole mass spectrometers because of their strength in quantitative applications.[32] In the regulatory considerations for these analyses, as LDTs, a common set of parameters should be examined, and these include linearity, intraday and interday precision and accuracy, sensitivity, selectivity, stability, interferences, matrix effects, carryover, and a comparison with a reference method. There are several regulatory standards and benchmarks for these parameters (Clinical and Laboratory Standard Institute, College of American Pathology, FDA Bioanalytical Guidance for Industry,[33] and so forth), although no single set of guidelines is universally accepted for these LDTs. The other application is MALDI-TOF MS for microbial identification, which represents an FDA-approved untargeted analysis, where, rather than a specific analyte being interrogated, the entire spectrum is analyzed for numerous analytes. This scenario matches more closely the current implementation of most ambient MS methods that use untargeted analysis of the lipidome, as discussed earlier. However, in the case of the approved MALDI-TOF MS test, the analytes are multiple microbial proteins, which are then used to identify and speciate the bacteria or fungi based on their similarity to a validated database of MS profiles. There are currently 2 FDA-approved platforms for microbial identification in the United States: the Biotyper (Bruker)[26] and the VITEK MS[27] (Biomerieux). These platforms both use comparable TOF mass analyzers but different statistical approaches to classify the isolates. In the approval process for microbial identification using MALDI-TOF-MS, both commercial entities sought and achieved FDA approval through a 510(k) Substantial Equivalence Determination, comparing their approaches with other FDA-approved identification techniques, such as 16S ribosomal RNA sequencing in the case of bacterial identification and Internal transcribed spacer or D1/D2 sequencing for fungal identification. However, one challenge with translating this to cancer is that there are no universal gold standard platforms already approved by the FDA. Most cancer diagnoses still require expert histopathologic review. Therefore, using a substantial equivalence determination will be difficult to achieve. Nonetheless, the fact that different statistical approaches are both approved by the FDA to perform the same task of microbial speciation is an important detail when considering the regulatory hurdles for ambient methods that use a variety of data analysis and statistical approaches[7,11,12,24,34–46] (eg, least absolute shrinkage and selection operator, principal component/linear discriminant analysis, partial least square discriminant analysis). Therefore, any statistical approach that can accurately and reproducibly differentiate tumor from nontumor tissue may be acceptable if it achieves the clinical diagnostic goals it promises.

Although targeted and untargeted analyses vary widely in their approach and requirements, they both share the common element of needing to meet specific benchmarks or criteria to be used in the clinical space. Although there are no widely accepted guidelines for validation of clinical ambient MS methods, it seems reasonable to imagine that the same approach that is applied to LC-MS/MS could be applied to ambient MS using QC samples. Ambient MS approaches may be in either the targeted category, wherein, for example, presence of a well-characterized oncometabolite is used to indicate disease, or the untargeted category, where overall changes in the spectral patterns are used to indicate disorder, depending on the analytes used and the diagnostic goal. Although this article touches on the relevant parameters, there are a few particular parameters, including carryover, stability, repeatability, surrounding environment, and matrix effects, that must be controlled and are worth discussing generally here because of their relevance and greater impact.

STANDARDIZING THE WORKFLOW FOR VALIDATION OF AMBIENT MASS SPECTROMETRY METHODS

Table 1 summarizes the considerations reviewed earlier, relevant to various ambient MS use case scenarios. This table further lists some of the broad challenges faced in adapting validation guidelines available for targeted MS approaches to ambient methods, where predictions are performed through untargeted, multivariate assessments of MS profiles. This table provides a reasonably broad summary of factors that must be taken into consideration for ambient MS, alongside challenges and solutions as a quick reference guide, and additional details to expand on some of the concepts introduced in this table are provided later. Although the absence of a harmonized workflow for validation of untargeted MS methods leaves many details to users to define first, helpful parallels can be drawn from the emergent field of agricultural product authentication (or food fraud), where molecular fingerprinting methods[47] and untargeted MS approaches[48] have gained popularity to detect nongenuine products. Analytical studies of agricultural products, initially only focused on QC using targeted methods to identify select contaminants or adulterants, have now been expanded to include authenticity evaluations to detect economically motivated adulterations (EMA) in food products using untargeted methods.[49] At present, published recommendations for harmonization of validation workflows of untargeted methods for EMA detection using a generalized approach are available.[29] These guidelines bear much relevance to the framework required to further validate ambient MS methods for cancer research.

By extrapolation from the recommendations referenced earlier for EMA detection, a robust multivariate data model established from a clearly defined and studied reference dataset must first be subjected to internal validation using a suitable cross-validation method, such as an iterative leave-out test, and then evaluated through external validation against a distinct secondary test dataset, preferably in a blind

Table 1

Regulatory consideration and recommendations for validation of ambient mass spectrometry assays

Important Elements	Considerations for Ambient MS	Challenges	Solutions and Recommendations
Intended use	Establish the intended clinical use	Pathology determination using untargeted analysis of ambient MS spectra is one of many use scenarios	In case of a targeted approach, guidelines reported for LDTs based on MS are best followed. Harmonized validation guidelines for untargeted approaches must first be developed
Precision	Measure assay output (eg, lesion classification as malignant vs normal) within each run/batch and across different days and score for concordance of predictions from each measurement. A reference specimen containing malignancy should be used	Reference materials such as tissue homogenates may offer good control over specimen stability issues but fail to address tissue molecular heterogeneities that could influence precision assessments. At present, no MS-centric SOPs for generalized reference material storage and analysis exist, and various methods require different degrees of operator manual intervention, potentially creating biases. Case-independent metrics for good-quality mass spectra do not exist. At present, no recommendations with respect to user qualifications in performing high-complexity assays exist	MS profiles of commonly occurring elements that persist in the specimen, such as stroma, should be cataloged and included in the analysis. SOPs for storage of reference material based on LC-MS/MS profiling of lipidome/analyte of interest using a high-resolution mass analyzer and storage guidelines that reproduce spectral/retention patterns most closely resembling fresh tissue must be established. In the case of a clinical specimen, as opposed to cases where tissue homogenates are used, the specimen must be inspected by a pathologist to validate presence of normal levels of heterogeneity common to clinical specimens. The influence of heterogeneity may be assessed by performing multiple samplings across the specimen and scoring for convergence. Internal metrics for relevant spectral features (abundance, complexity) that are required for

(continued on next page)

Table 1
(continued)

Important Elements	Considerations for Ambient MS	Challenges	Solutions and Recommendations
			classification of MS readout using the specimen under study must be established. Ideally, poor-quality spectra that do not meet the established criteria should not be included in the classification. Inspection of multivariate loading plots for the presence of strongly differentiating ions (ie, tissue classifying markers) can be used to verify spectral complexity and suitability of said measurement. The authors encourage experimental measurements to be performed by more than 1 user, with variance in results documented
Accuracy	Measure assay output (eg, lesion classification as malignant vs normal) against anatomic or molecular pathology gold standards. A reference tissue containing malignancy should be used	See above, as discussed for precision	See above, as discussed for precision. The authors encourage accuracy measurements to be performed using blind tests where the operator of MS is blinded to the correct classification of the samples. We also encourage use of both control (healthy) and malignant specimens. This assessment should use the same multivariate analysis platform/algorithm intended for clinical use, because cross-platform variations are currently poorly understood

Reportable range	Measure assay output (eg, lesion classification as malignant vs normal) against anatomic or molecular pathology gold standards using a reference sample such as tissue homogenate containing different amounts of malignancy (eg, percentage of cancer cells)	Presence of tissue heterogeneity can influence the reportable range, herein defined as assay tolerance to certain percentage of interfering heterogeneity signal, to generate output consistent with pathology gold standards	Artificially created average spectra by mixing known percentages of pure signals (eg, healthy and malignant) can be used to examine the performance of the multivariate method in a reportable to avoid the pathology/disease rules range. This method ties in with the concept of clinical sensitivity where anatomic pathology offers sensitivity on the single-cell resolution, not matched by all ambient MS methods currently available
Reference interval	Establish assay output variance (eg, lesion classification as malignant vs normal) across a sufficiently large population of healthy individuals and correlate to anatomic or molecular pathology gold standards	The diverse nature of multivariate statistical analysis methods used prevent prescription of a one-size-fits-all method of variance measurement across healthy cohorts	Power calculations may be performed while considering existing knowledge of the extent of pathologic or molecular heterogeneity in a given population. This extent may be assessed via anatomic or molecular pathology methods, performed over the desired clinical reportable range
Analytical sensitivity	Establish analytical sensitivity by combining the recommendations above on precision, applied within the determined reportable range	See above, as discussed for precision and reportable range	See above, as discussed for precision and reportable range
Analytical specificity	Establish analytical specificity by combining the recommendations above on accuracy, applied within the determined reportable range	See above, as discussed for accuracy and reportable range	See above, as discussed for accuracy and reportable range
Sample or reagent stability	Examine sample stability by performing time-dependent measurements of the assay output (and freeze/thaw cycles, if applicable)	See above as discussed for precision and accuracy	See above as discussed for precision and accuracy

(continued on next page)

Table 1
(continued)

Important Elements	Considerations for Ambient MS	Challenges	Solutions and Recommendations
Process and environmental factors	Examine carryover between assay runs/ different specimen measurements using, for example, normal and malignant specimens analyzed in tandem. Assess the assay output against collection by different users	See above, as discussed for precision and accuracy. In addition, an environmental human factor assessment of the tool in the context of intended use considering other compliances required (eg, electrical, patient safety, operating room use compliance using national and international guidelines) must be used	See above, as discussed for precision and accuracy. Because currently mass spectrometers are implemented only transiently in clinical settings or within an operating theater for trial purposes only, a detailed human factor assessment with an environmental use concern focus associated with long-term widespread use in light of compliances required must be conducted. In this realm, airflow disturbances and treatment of aerosolized material not taken up by the spectrometer and released into the operating room must be considered for safety implications. Likewise, the impact of any mitigation strategy managing the spread of aerosolized particles on MS signal stability must be determined
Lot-to-lot variability in consumables	Examine lot-to-lot variability of solvents for ambient MS methods that use solvents by measuring the assay output using standard specimens across different solvent batches. For ambient methods that do not use solvents, develop own process for QC (eg, laser fiber transmission)	Not all MS-based methods use solvents. Probe components such as laser fiber or electrocautery blades should undergo normal QC assessments for performance, and then be reassessed for stable MS signal. The standard QC protocols for these tools do not necessarily review performance for stable MS signal	The authors recommend evaluating each new batch with a precision measurement, as discussed above

Surrounding environment influence	Keep the environment surrounding the source as constant as possible	Ambient MS operates in open air; fluctuations of ambient conditions (temperature, humidity, air conditioning changes) can lead to variances in MS results	The authors recommend usage of devices to control humidity and temperature of the room. Keep the door closed and avoid fast movements of personnel. Where engineering controls are not possible, at least document the variable factors such as temperature, humidity, usage, and their influence on assay results
Drift in instrument response/ calibration errors	Routinely monitor the calibration of the MS analyzer	High-resolution mass spectrometers (TOF and orbitraps) may be affected by drifts in calibration for a few ppm	Calibrate every day and use lock-mass systems. Keep the temperature of the room constant. Understand and document the influence of drift on the precision and accuracy of predictions and the performance of the multivariate platform used
Carryover	Routinely monitor carryover between the runs	Presence of tissue residues is possible on the source probe, transport tube, and inside the MS inlet. Routine cleaning of the inlet may not require breaking vacuum, but cleaning the contamination inside the instrument may require pump-down, affecting the duty cycle	Monitor carryover by running a blank between each batch of samples or independent runs. Establish the frequency of inlet cleaning if necessary. Resort to having a second instrument on standby to reduce downtime in case deep cleaning beyond the inlet is required after some use
System or instrumentation variability	Follow MS manufacturing guidelines for detector setup. Develop own process for ionization interface performance measurements and evaluation of performance. Develop own protocol for desorption source performance. Variabilities can be examined based on the recommendations provided above for precision using a suitable reference tissue material	Many ambient sources are still undergoing reengineering for improvements in performance. As such, a large number of variables are expected to influence performance variability (eg, laser power, alignment, tissue water content [for infrared systems], cautery blade geometry). An assessment of variability should use same system components as used in the assay	The authors recommend evaluating variability with a precision measurement, as discussed above

(continued on next page)

Table 1
(continued)

Important Elements	Considerations for Ambient MS	Challenges	Solutions and Recommendations
Clinical sensitivity	Determine false-negative rates, preferably in a blind test/ring (multisite; multiuser) tests	High rates of false-negatives are possible when the multivariate model dataset is capturing insufficient variability/heterogeneity in the samples	Populate the multivariate modeling datasets with as many heterogenous samples as possible, as per power calculations, and obtain an understanding of the intrinsic biological variability within the patient population. Some multivariate methods perform better than others when intersample variability is less than intrasample variability, or vice versa. See the challenges and recommendations provided above for precision measurements
Clinical specificity	Determine false-positive rates, preferably in a blind test/ring (multisite; multiuser) tests	High rates of false-positives are possible when the model dataset is overly sensitive to heterogeneity factors that are present in biological tissue but are not necessarily associated with the disease state	Refine the multivariate modeling dataset to find the right balance (as per blind sample validations) between capturing heterogeneity in tissue as well as in disease states. See the recommendations provided above for precision and for clinical sensitivity with respect to understanding intersample/intrasample variabilities and their influence on the performance of multivariate prediction methods. Also, see below as recommended for automation of acquisition and results

Special safety controls	Establish and follow guidelines that ensure safe use in patients or provide compliance with respect to the environment in which the tools may be used. The text provides more information on some elements with respect to human factor assessment using simulated use scenarios, user/operator qualifications, use hazards and compliances (IEC, ISO), and adverse effect traceability documents as well as maintenance and operational manuals	Because MS methodologies can integrate within various clinical workflows and be used by a diverse group of operators with vastly varying training backgrounds, a one-size-fits-all recommendation cannot be made	Intended use must first be defined to determine a comprehensive list of special controls that are relevant with respect to both the environment at which the tool is intended for use and with respect to the qualifications/training the intended users must possess. Patient safety is of paramount importance. Therefore, any method used for in vivo assessments is expected to be safe for such use and provide risk assessment and adverse effect traceability documentations that detail risk mitigation strategies
Assay controls	Combining the recommendations above on precision and instrument variability, establish guidelines for spectral robustness, mass accuracy (eg, effect of mass drift/day-to-day variations, and signal suppression)	See above, as discussed for precision and instrument variability	See above, as discussed for precision and instrument variability
Document control	Within the determined intended clinical use, proceed to establish SOPs as well as workflow documents. Taking the results of human factor assessments into consideration, establish appropriate user qualification and training guidelines commensurate with the degree of expertise required for potential manual interventions if necessary	The performance of each assay is highly dependent on the desorption source and the instrument on which it is validated. Therefore, implementation on any new instrument or interface requires revising said SOPs	Establish these documents once the intended use scenario is determined

(continued on next page)

Table 1
(continued)

Important Elements	Considerations for Ambient MS	Challenges	Solutions and Recommendations
Automated acquisition and results	To reduce sources of variation, automated collection of data and MS profile matching is highly desirable	In the absence of automated analysis, the results will be influenced by user mistakes or bias. However, multivariate methods may overfit the data	Incorporate as much automation as possible but allow access to raw data and adjustable parameters to verify sources of assay output variations or failures. A combination of supervised and unsupervised multivariate methods can be used to ascertain statistically significant alterations to the spectral profiles without concerns that overfitting is taking place. Also, see above for clinical sensitivity and specificity and recommendations provided therein. A clear data-independent definition of a good-quality spectrum is required in automated methods to prevent a garbage-in, garbage-out–type scenario

This table summarizes important regulatory considerations and challenges associated with adapting these common regulatory understandings to ambient MS methods and includes additional recommendations. This table only serves as a preliminary guide, and may not be comprehensive or complete in its contents, especially given the variations in permutations of possible clinical applications that may be envisioned for ambient MS. The considerations provided in this table have been put together using a disease (cancer or malignant) scenario. Not all items and components may be relevant to other envisioned applications.

Abbreviation: IEC, International Electrotechnical Commission; ISO, International Organization for Standardization; SOPs, standard operating procedures.

fashion. Thorough validation for clinical use further requires a high degree of result reproducibility across different laboratories, instruments, and operators. To the best of our knowledge, nontargeted ambient MS methods to date have been mainly laboratory developed with few attempts to determine interlaboratory reproducibility, as exemplified by these reports.[50–52] Although harmonized guidelines to validate ambient MS methods are yet to be drafted, the number of researchers using untargeted ambient MS methods in cancer research is growing and is further expected to create a demand pull for devising validation guidelines. Here, close communications with clinical chemists who are familiar with both regulatory guidelines and principles of LDT and analytical reproducibility and robustness is expected to greatly benefit this endeavor.

Sample Allocation Strategy and Power Calculations

Power calculation tools[53] to calculate appropriate numbers of samples[54] and the minimum number of samples suitable for multivariate data models have been reported.[55] Integration of multisite data and multiplatform data, and subsequent evaluation of the performance of data fused across different platforms or sites,[56] is expected to further assess the robustness of a proposed validation workflow. Capturing biological variance[57] is an important aspect of experimental design,[58] and replicates must be included to minimize uncontrolled variations seen across the larger population.[59] Methods reported in the literature to date may not offer the robustness needed for widespread clinical accredited use and should not be used as gold standards on the grounds of having been peer reviewed, especially when it comes down to sample numbers. In our opinion, most published studies so far have used limited numbers of samples to validate a proof of concept. Here, the recent approvals of a registered clinical trial to assess the efficacy of iKnife in breast surgery are highly encouraging (NCT03432429). Along the same lines, ring trails for multisite validation, where the same agents are sent to different laboratories for analysis and reporting, are important to assess the reliability of nontargeted diagnostic approaches across different laboratories. Although first-level (or higher) identification of markers responsible for classifications according to the criteria proposed by Standard Initiative in Metabolomics[60,61] is not per se required, an identified marker orthogonally validated or known to be involved in a disease process, as an example, would certainly boost users' confidence in the validation workflow.

Sample and Analyte Stability

Specimen or analyte stability is another important consideration with any clinical assay. In LC-MS/MS methods, typical stability studies include autosampler, 24-hour room temperature, freeze-thaw, as well as short-term and long-term and stock stability studies, in case samples are being stored before analysis.[33] However, like carryover, stability studies should cover the conditions most relevant to the collection, transport, and specimen storage, if any, before analysis. Because of wide use of tissue lipids in ambient MS methods discussed earlier, specimen stability is of paramount importance in the analysis of ex vivo fresh or frozen tissue specimens. Because lipidome undergoes drastic changes during cell death[62] and because of storage conditions,[63] the consequence of tissue handling on sample adequacy for ambient MS must be evaluated thoroughly.[63] For example, false-positives may arise in clinical assays designed to determine the degree of necrosis within a tumor based on tissue ceramides[6,64] because of improper handling or storage.[62,63]

Tissue Preservation During the Ambient Mass Spectrometry Analysis

The amount of material removed by different ambient desorption sources creates a further divide in the degree of depth profiling offered by various ambient MS sampling methods. Some ambient methods form true surface sampling tools that permit downstream histopathologic assessments of the same tissue piece after MS analysis,[65] whereas others permanently remove tissue and thus rely exclusively on adjacent tissue for histopathologic assessment. These attributes are particularly important to consider when devising validation strategies in cases where there is a requirement for tissue preservation for additional testing (eg, genetic, histologic) following mass spectrometric analysis, or in cases where the MS probe is used for the purposes of QC on a specimen to be subjected to downstream clinical analysis work flows (eg, biopsy adequacy). An inherent complication arises where tissue heterogeneity, affecting the MS profiles, changes on the length scale of ambient measurements or even sectioning, rendering adjacent tissue evaluations irrelevant for cross-validation purposes. Here, the development of gentle ambient sampling methods is highly encouraging.[14]

Instrumental Drift and Use of Quality Control Samples to Monitor Instrumental Performances

The transient nature of signal in some ambient MS methods, especially those created by uncontrolled aerosolization methods, has created an impetus for the use of TOF instruments that offer rapid scan times over a wide mass range. Therefore, the issue of instrumental drift and its implications on accurate profiling, relevant to many of the reported applications, becomes significant in the context of any future targeted analyses, especially quantitative analyses. Here, the ambient methods that rely on solvents for extraction or improved desorption allow fusion of lock-mass reference compounds for real-time correction of potential instrumental drifts.[66] However, in practice, most real-time ambient analysis reports have used spectral binning[7,11,12] as opposed to centroid fits, and this to some extent may accommodate minor instrumental drifts. Therefore, the trade-off between analytical sensitivity and specificity that arises because of spectral binning for rapid results using the entire mass range must be taken into consideration in any future adaptation of ambient methods using TOF instruments for quantitative targeted detection of analytes. Reproducibility and repeatability may be determined by using QC or reference samples.

Carryover

One additional consideration is carryover. In addition to the standard carryover issues that come with any MS method, for ambient methods there is an additional challenge in that the sample probe is often in near, or direct, contact with the tissue being analyzed. A small fragment of tissue getting caught on the tip of the probe could lead to persistent detection of that analyte or to the suppression of other analytes, leading to false-positive or false-negative results. This possibility has considerable clinical ramifications because surgeons could be making clinical decisions based on these results. There are some platforms, for example, in the case of liquid extraction surface analysis, where a disposable tip and nanoelectrospray nozzle are used to limit any carryover.[67] Ambient MS methods that use suction to transport vaporized/desorbed tissue molecules to the ionization interface and mass analyzer are not immune to this. However, they provide an opportunity to verify presence of carryover by performing a rapid blank measurement from a tip not exposed to surgical specimen as a control.

Matrix Effects

Matrix effects are an important consideration in any MS application, but particularly when gentle ionization techniques such as electrospray ionization (ESI) and desorption ESI (DESI) are used. Although both are excellent ionization techniques compatible with many biological analytes and matrices, one of their primary shortcomings is ion suppression as the molecules in the spray are competing for charge.[68] Signal suppression caused by matrix elements is an even greater concern when it comes to ambient approaches in which the analytes are not cleaned up or separated chromatographically before analysis. It is conceivable that ambient MS sources that use solvents/analyte interactions to promote ionization through an ESI-like process will suffer from ion suppression effects, requiring the same rigor in selection of solvent matrix and analysis of lot-to-lot variations using reference compounds, as done in compliant LC-MS/MS assays. Although the notion of matrix may be interpreted differently in other ambient methods, its influence on the MS signal should be investigated closely. For example, ambient sources that use water molecules, which are abundant in biological tissues, to drive desorption (such as those based on infrared lasers[7,12]) may show intrasample or intersample variances in performance or desorption efficiencies based on water content variations within a tissue.

Clinical Sensitivity and Mass Spectrometry Spatial Resolution

In the context of future implementation of ambient MS in clinical workflows, the issue of clinical sensitivity becomes of paramount importance. Histopathology methods can offer sensitivities at the single-cell level. As the MS readout reflects on population averaging of signal at the interrogated pixel, the impact of spatial resolution for applications such as margin assessment of highly infiltrative tumors cannot be discounted. However, many of the point sampling studies have focused on interrogation of tumor cores (largely devoid of significant heterogeneities on the length scale of pixels examined) for the purpose of rapid tumor type identification from m/z profile matching against preestablished (and validated with pathology gold standards) tumor type m/z libraries. Handheld MS desorption probes have shown utility for examining both in vivo and ex vivo tissue samples, and range widely in their abilities and performance metrics such as spatial resolution, reported analytical (or clinical) sensitivity, specificity, and degree of invasiveness/destructiveness to the specimens analyzed.

Controlled Surroundings to Minimize Impact on Signal Reproducibility

The aerosol pickup inlets of ambient MS sources are engineered to work optimally under atmospheric pressure and room temperature conditions. As such, possible fluctuations in ambient conditions such as changes in the temperature, movement of the operators, humidity, and air flow modifications may lead to variations in MS signal. For regulatory assessments, documenting the effect of environmental factors on performance may be important. Although creating enclosures to shield the pickup source against environmental variations such as movement of operators and airflow can be incorporated in some applications, uncontrolled aerosolization of pathogen-containing specimens, brought about by ambient MS sources, may pose an additional safety risk. Although samplings could take place inside a biological safety cabinet or in the presence of suction devices to minimize the spread of aerosols generated during in vivo ambient MS, the impact of all such devices on MS signal reproducibility must be documented. Although strategies to normalize data to account for variations in signal strength have been used in multivariate assessments, the sensitivity of multivariate predictions to signal-to-noise fluctuations that could arise because of environmental factors affecting collection or desorption efficiencies is poorly under-stood and must be systematically evaluated.

Automated Acquisition and Processing of Data

To further reduce sources of variation, automated collection of data, preprocessing of the spectra (alignment, background removal, deisotoping, normalization) and statisti-cal predictions with profile matching against validated m/z profile libraries unified in an accredited automated system is highly desirable. However, the ability to access and evaluate raw data to better understand the origin of classification failures has been a key aspect to the development of ambient methods so far. Additional model-independent metrics for data QC must be incorporated in any automated setup to avoid a garbage-in, garbage-out scenario. The degree of automation will have an impact on the user qualification and training required, and is also important for regu-latory approval.

ADDITIONAL REQUIREMENTS ASSOCIATED WITH DEPLOYMENT WITHIN A CLINICAL SETTING

The versatility of ambient MS sources in terms of their potential to integrate with the variety of clinical workflows summarized earlier and reviewed in **Fig. 1** translates to different types of regulatory and safety compliance considerations that must be dis-cussed. These requirements are not only tied into the device's mode of use (ex vivo, in vivo), the probe's degree of destructiveness to the specimens, and whether clinical decisions are made based on device's output but also include additional re-quirements associated with the clinical setting in which the device is intended for use. For example, en route to adoption, handheld ambient MS probes that come into contact with patients within an operating room (OR) for the purpose of clinical de-cision making must satisfy all the requirements of (1) a robust clinical assay, (2) demonstrated safety for use in or near patients, and (3) compliance with OR use re-quirements (eg, wipeable surfaces; no disruption of OR airflow; and manageable foot-print, noise, and heat dissipation profiles). To simplify some of these requirements, remote imaging applications,[39] or near-patient analysis protocols have been envi-sioned[69] that involve, for example, having the mass analyzer on standby outside the operating theater or extending the connection between the imaging interface and the mass analyzer such that only the former is present inside the operating theater to minimize air flow disturbance or noise or heat pollution inside the OR arising from the inner workings of the mass analyzer itself.

AMBIENT MASS SPECTROMETRY USE CASES IN THE CLINICAL DOMAIN

Clinical diagnostic opportunities for ambient ionization MS can be broadly divided into in vivo and ex vivo applications (**Fig. 1**). In vivo applications refer to those that involve direct in situ sampling of the patient, whereas ex vivo applications involve sampling specimens after they have been removed from the patient. Ex vivo applications can be separated into those in which a clinical decision is being made (eg, presence of tu-mor or pathogen) and those that are primarily considering adequacy of the sample for additional downstream analyses. Although the latter have a significant impact (deci-sion to resample), it is arguably less consequential than making a clinical diagnosis. Both in vivo and ex vivo approaches present benefits and challenges and invoke com-mon as well as unique regulatory concerns. There are many other ambient MS appli-cations, most notably in the forensics, food safety, or environmental fields,[15,70–73] which also require thorough and thoughtful regulatory considerations, but those are

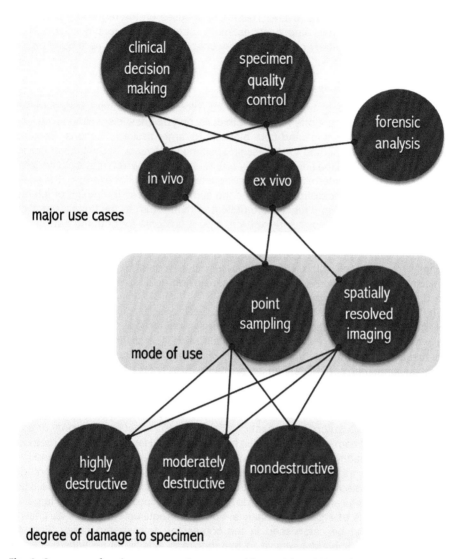

Fig. 1. Summary of major use scenarios reported for ambient MS applications. In general, applications involve cases where clinical decision is made using in vivo or ex vivo tissue or no clinical decision is made, such as applications of ambient MS for specimen QC (eg, biopsy adequacy) or forensics. Forensics applications are not discussed further in this article. For biopsy adequacy, it is important that the chosen MS method does not drastically alter the specimen to the point of hampering downstream conventional analyses. Here, the rapid readout attribute of ambient MS method is used to confirm presence of disorder within the specimen and accordingly obtain subsequent samples in case of inadequacy. For all other applications that involve in vivo analysis, the ambient MS probe should satisfy safety requirements and the device should conform to specific site requirements, such as wipeable surfaces for use in the operating theater and exhaust/heat/noise outputs that are within relevant guidelines. MS methods can be used in both point sampling and imaging modes and possess varying degrees of destructiveness to the specimen. The degree of specimen destruction during ambient MS sampling may in turn create additional requirements of

outside of the scope of this review. This article focuses on the regulatory considerations for ex vivo and in vivo applications, moving from less to more invasive/consequential applications. Many of the regulatory conditions discussed here build on the concepts discussed earlier.

Sample Adequacy Studies

Surgeons, cytopathologists, interventional radiologists, and other proceduralists, such as endoscopists, are often tasked with collecting diagnostic specimens, ranging from fine-needle aspirations and core biopsies to larger tissue resections. Because there is no bona fide method for assessing specimen adequacy at the time of collection, it is often not until the final pathology report is available, which may be days later, that the specimen is determined to be inadequate because of, for example, the specimen only containing necrotic tissue, or if the sampling misses the region of interest entirely. This situation may require the patient to then return to the hospital or clinic and undergo a repeat biopsy or reexcision, a poor outcome for both the patient and the diagnostic team. This problem is common in prostate biopsies, where the biopsy needle can deviate or bend and miss the lesion.[74] Therefore, the ability to assess these samples for adequacy at the time of biopsy would be a great benefit for patients and clinicians. The same issue exists for breast cancer, where a significant number of biopsied specimen do not contain disease.[75]

Although no clinical decision is being made, the central question is whether the collected specimen is adequate for further assessment through the clinical workflow. So, what are the critical or assay characteristics when it comes to sample adequacy? The first and foremost is a determination on what defines an adequate specimen. An adequate specimen can be defined as the minimum quantity and quality of specimen needed to make a diagnosis. Therefore, a chemical signature must be developed for each clinical tissue to include both the presence and/or absence of particular analytes. As discussed earlier, sample handling affects the MS profile for accurate assessment of adequacy, and therefore the impact of MS sampling on specimen integrity or adequacy for downstream assessment must be investigated. Here, ambient MS methods with their rapid readout attributes, especially those that offer high sensitivity and less destruction to the specimen outside the sampling zone,[14,65] offer a definite advantage, ensuring the biopsied sample contains the lesion in question for subsequent conventional histopathology analysis. For any downstream application that requires targeted molecular analysis of a particular analyte, additional requirements, such as analyte stability, must first be established in the context of downstream assay. For MS methods that are highly destructive to the specimen, additional sections/pieces of the specimen must be considered for downstream assessments. Here, extensive heterogeneity on the length scale of pixels examined may make parallel section examinations less attractive to report on MS readout of adequacy. It is also important to consider how clinical samples deemed inadequate by ambient analysis methods will be handled; will they be discarded altogether or kept for future reexaminations? The impact of this on patient well-being and attitude to the test should be considered.

---

serial section preservation for validation, record keeping or additional downstream analyses, and parallel initial integration into existing clinical workflows. For example, when sampling with a nondestructive ambient MS probe results in little structural or molecular damage to the specimen and compatibility with, for example, histopathologic staining exists, initial integration into existing workflows can take place seamlessly without concerns for sample preservation for orthogonal validation or downstream use.

Ex Vivo Clinical Diagnostic Studies

In addition to sample adequacy, ex vivo diagnostic approaches have been developed using ambient MS as described earlier. In this case, the tissue of interest is excised from the patient and analyzed by ambient MS ex vivo, similar to the frozen section procedure in pathology. One of the advantages is that this method is faster than the frozen section procedure, which involves transporting the sample to the frozen section room, freezing the sample, sectioning it in a cryostat, followed by hematoxylin-eosin (H&E) staining and review by an experienced pathologist. In ex vivo ambient MS approaches, the sample can be analyzed immediately after it is excised from the patient, even in the OR, and with little or no sample preparation, which can cut down turnaround time (TAT) significantly compared with frozen sections. In addition to TAT improvements, another key advantage of using MS is the ability to assess the tissue based on its chemical signature, rather than relying only on histopathologic changes. Multiple groups have shown not only that, using ambient ionization MS lipidomic approaches, tissues can be classified as benign versus malignant but also that cancers can be further subclassified using lipid signatures alone. A recent example of this is subgrouping of pediatric medulloblastoma cancers into their 4 clinically relevant and prognostically important molecular subgroups[76,77] using ambient PIRL-MS with 10-second readout.[7] Medulloblastoma cells are morphologically indistinguishable with simple H&E staining, and classification uses either genetic or immunohistochemistry methods.[78] However, despite these advantages, there are some limitations and important considerations when using these approaches.

Analyte stability is an important consideration when considering ex vivo diagnostic approaches because there are time-dependent chemical and biological changes that occur after a specimen is removed from the body that can affect MS analysis, as discussed earlier.[63] Chemically, there are certain metabolites and lipids that oxidize or can break down when exposed to air or the surface in which the sample is being analyzed.[79] Proteins can also be degraded through proteolysis. However, more concerning are the biological changes that occur. Because the tissue is no longer perfused once ex vivo, there are several metabolic changes that occur in the cell, including posttranslational modifications to enzymes involved in energy metabolism as well as upregulation or downregulation of signaling molecules.[62,64,80,81] There are approaches that have been used to mitigate or at least decrease these changes. The most common approach is to rapidly snap freeze the specimen in liquid nitrogen, for example, thereby quenching the metabolic activity of the cells. The cells generally have to be thawed to analyze and it has been shown that metabolic activity can return during the thawing cycle. Therefore, another approach that has been used is thermal inactivation of enzymes using either laboratory-developed or commercially available platforms.[82] This process inactivates metabolic enzymes as well as proteases and lipases, which reduces degradation of metabolites, proteins, and lipids, respectively, and more faithfully represents the biochemical state of the tissue at the time it was collected. However, either approach will slow down the TAT and may render the method unacceptable for its intended clinical use. Therefore, a careful balance between sample stability and TAT must be considered, and the impact of thermal inactivation on ambient MS profiles of lipids must first be understood.

Another important consideration with any of these approaches is sensitivity caused by the intrinsic heterogeneity of biological specimens or degree of infiltration of lesion into normal tissue. One of the approaches to performing ex vivo analysis is by creating a squash prep, where the tissue is pressed between 2 glass slides before analysis.[8,10,83] Although this provides a fast approach, one important element that is lost is spatial resolution or spatial integrity of the tissue. Because of the heterogenous nature of neoplastic and infectious processes, this loss of spatial resolution can lead to a concomitant decrease in sensitivity caused by mixing of normal and malignant tissue. To overcome this, a sample can be cryosectioned and DESI-MS imaging can be performed on the tissue, which is rastered in 2 dimensions, resulting in a chemical image. This method provides better spatial resolution and, along with this, better sensitivity because the sample is not mixed. However, it is challenging to achieve rapid scan times without sacrificing sensitivity, especially for large pieces of tissue.

In Vivo Clinical Diagnostic Studies

Perhaps some of the most exciting applications for ambient MS involves the in vivo applications. Of course, as with any method, the standard assay characteristics and parameters apply, along with the ambient-specific parameters described earlier for the ex vivo approaches. However, there are additional considerations specific for in vivo applications, most notably that the probe and device are safe for the patient as well as other use site compatibility considerations. The 2 most mature in vivo approaches are arguably REIMS (iKnife)[11] and the MasSpec Pen,[14] although a variety of other laser-based methods are also being introduced for in vivo work.[84] REIMS uses the smoke from an electrocautery tool (or recently other surgical lasers[24]) for MS analysis, whereas the MasSpec Pen[14] uses a new tool in which a water droplet carried to the tissue surface serves as a solvent to solubilize tissue-classifying lipids and metabolites for the purpose of determining tissue type or detection of the presence of a tumor.[14] Regardless of what approach is taken to sample the body, what makes in vivo approaches particularly exciting is the ability to sample the tissue in situ. This ability provides surgeons with real-time chemical feedback to guide surgical decision making. Another advantage of in vivo approaches is that it minimizes or even completely avoids the post-resection changes that may occur in the tissue, thereby providing a chemical signature that more faithfully represents the physiologic state of the tissue, reducing the need for more extensive stability studies.

There are some challenges as well, most notably regarding patient safety. Unlike ex vivo approaches, in vivo approaches require manipulation of some interface within the patient. In the case of the REIMS, the use of an electrocautery tool overcomes the requirement of introducing a new medical or sample device because these are already used in surgery. In contrast, the MasSpec Pen[14] uses biocompatible materials but, because this is a new device, it is likely to require the same regulatory and safety requirements as any other surgical tool. As detailed earlier, additional considerations exist beyond safety for in vivo clinical diagnostics, and many of these relate to use site compatibility. These considerations include that the apparatus, including the mass analyzer and the probe, have an acceptable footprint; wipeable surface; and do not produce noise, heat, or airflow disturbances that would interfere with OR conditions or safety, or affect the sterile field. Further, the electrical and exhaust requirements must be compatible with site requirements. The degree of automation and the need to access and evaluate raw data directly affect use scenario definitions. Here, educational and experience requirements for performing high-complexity assays, training and competency, and evidence of compliance documents must be considered as well.

SUMMARY

Ambient MS methods offer rapid (within seconds) access to clinically important information such as tissue disease state. The reported proof-of-principle studies have attested to the power of these techniques in accelerating disease state determination without extensive preanalytical preparations, and accuracy on the order of 98% or greater in some cases has been reported. Although rigorous multisite validation of ambient methods using large patient pools is beginning to emerge, the recent FDA approvals of untargeted MALDI-TOF MS approaches for microbial identification using different statistical algorithms can serve as a positive sign that regulatory approvals on the grounds of performance and reproducibility can be granted in the absence of fully characterizing the nature of disorder-determining molecules. The approval of an untargeted MS technique, mentioned earlier, based on reproducibility of validated predictions can be likened to the journey taken by anatomic pathology and its quintessential role in clinical decision making, now extensively validated against outcomes. Although the extent to which the speedy delivery of tissue disease state information with ambient methods may alter the clinical course of conventional treatments is yet to be evaluated and validated against outcomes, ambient MS methods that use sampling probes already validated for use in patients are expected to break through the regulatory barrier first.

CLINICS CARE POINTS

Pearls:

- Upon validation, a rapid delivery of objective clinical diagnoses at the bed side may be possible with ambient mass spectrometry.

Pitfalls:

- A harmonized performance validation including special safety and assay controls has not yet been developed.

ACKNOWLEDGMENTS

Ambient MS research in the Zarrine-Afsar group is supported by Princess Margaret Hospital and St Michael's Hospital Foundations, Canadian Institutes for Health Research (CIHR) Project Grant, and Natural Sciences and Engineering Research Council of Canada (NSERC) Discovery Grant programs.

DISCLOSURE

A.Z.-A. is a consultant with Point Surgical Inc.

REFERENCES

1. Ifa DR, Eberlin LS. Ambient ionization mass spectrometry for cancer diagnosis and surgical margin evaluation. Clin Chem 2016;62(1):111–23.
2. Santos CR, Schulze A. Lipid metabolism in cancer. FEBS J 2012;279(15): 2610–23.
3. Clark AR, Calligaris D, Regan MS, et al. Rapid discrimination of pediatric brain tumors by mass spectrometry imaging. J Neurooncol 2018;140(2):269–79.
4. Eberlin LS. DESI-MS imaging of lipids and metabolites from biological samples. Methods Mol Biol 2014;1198:299–311.
5. Pirro V, Jarmusch AK, Ferreira CR, et al. Ambient lipidomic analysis of brain tissue using desorption electrospray ionization (DESI) mass spectrometry. Neuromethods 2017;125:187–210.

6. Tata A, Woolman M, Ventura M, et al. Rapid detection of necrosis in breast cancer with desorption electrospray ionization mass spectrometry. Sci Rep 2016;6: 35374.

7. Woolman M, Kuzan-Fischer CM, Ferry I, et al. Picosecond infrared laser desorption mass spectrometry identifies medulloblastoma subgroups on intrasurgical timescales. Cancer Res 2019;79(9):2426–34.

8. Jarmusch AK, Pirro V, Baird Z, et al. Lipid and metabolite profiles of human brain tumors by desorption electrospray ionization-MS. Proc Natl Acad Sci U S A 2016; 113(6):1486–91.

9. Pirro V, Alfaro CM, Jarmusch AK, et al. Intraoperative assessment of tumor margins during glioma resection by desorption electrospray ionization-mass spectrometry. Proc Natl Acad Sci U S A 2017;114(26):6700–5.

10. Santagata S, Eberlin LS, Norton I, et al. Intraoperative mass spectrometry mapping of an onco-metabolite to guide brain tumor surgery. Proc Natl Acad Sci U S A 2014;111(30):11121–6.

11. Balog J, Sasi-Szabo L, Kinross J, et al. Intraoperative tissue identification using rapid evaporative ionization mass spectrometry. Sci Transl Med 2013;5(194): 194ra193.

12. Saudemont P, Quanico J, Robin YM, et al. Real-time molecular diagnosis of tumors using water-assisted laser desorption/ionization mass spectrometry technology. Cancer Cell 2018;34(5):840–51.e844.

13. Calligaris D, Norton I, Feldman DR, et al. Mass spectrometry imaging as a tool for surgical decision-making. J Mass Spectrom 2013;48(11):1178–87.

14. Zhang J, Rector J, Lin JQ, et al. Nondestructive tissue analysis for ex vivo and in vivo cancer diagnosis using a handheld mass spectrometry system. Sci Transl Med 2017;9(406):eaan3968.

15. Feider CL, Krieger A, DeHoog RJ, et al. Ambient ionization mass spectrometry: recent developments and applications. Anal Chem 2019;91(7):4266–90.

16. Takats Z, Strittmatter N, McKenzie JS. Ambient mass spectrometry in cancer research. Adv Cancer Res 2017;134:231–56.

17. Yannell KE, Smith K, Alfaro CM, et al. N-acetylaspartate and 2-hydroxyglutarate assessed in human brain tissue by mass spectrometry as Neuronal markers of oncogenesis. Clin Chem 2017;63(11):1766–7.

18. Koundouros N, Karali E, Tripp A, et al. Metabolic fingerprinting links oncogenic PIK3CA with enhanced arachidonic acid-derived eicosanoids. Cell 2020; 181(7):1596–611.e1527.

19. Woolman M, Qiu J, Kuzan-Fischer CM, et al. In situ tissue pathology from spatially encoded mass spectrometry classifiers visualized in real time through augmented reality. Chem Sci 2020;11(33):8723–35.

20. Tata A, Woolman M, Bluemke E, et al. Chapter 5 - ambient laser-based mass spectrometry analysis methods: a survey of core technologies and reported applications. In: Zaitsu K, editor. Ambient ionization mass spectrometry in Life Sciences. Amsterdam: Elsevier; 2020. p. 119–69.

21. Schafer KC, Balog J, Szaniszlo T, et al. Real time analysis of brain tissue by direct combination of ultrasonic surgical aspiration and sonic spray mass spectrometry. Anal Chem 2011;83(20):7729–35.

22. Takats Z, Wiseman JM, Gologan B, et al. Mass spectrometry sampling under ambient conditions with desorption electrospray ionization. Science 2004; 306(5695):471–3.

23. Sachfer KC, Szaniszlo T, Gunther S, et al. In situ, real-time identification of biological tissues by ultraviolet and infrared laser desorption ionization mass spectrometry. Anal Chem 2011;83(5):1632–40.

24. Genangeli M, Heeren RMA, Porta Siegel T. Tissue classification by rapid evaporative ionization mass spectrometry (REIMS): comparison between a diathermic knife and CO2 laser sampling on classification performance. Anal Bioanal Chem 2019;411(30):7943–55.

25. Zhang J, Sans M, Garza KY, et al. Mass spectrometry technologies to advance care for cancer patients in clinical and intraoperative Use. Mass Spectrom Rev 2020. https://doi.org/10.1002/mas.21664.

26. Available at: https://www.accessdata.fda.gov/cdrh_docs/reviews/K130831.pdf. Accessed March 30th, 2021.

27. Available at: https://www.accessdata.fda.gov/cdrh_docs/reviews/K162950.pdf.

28. Available at: https://www.fda.gov/media/89841/download.

29. USP Pharmacopeial Convention. Guidance on developing and validating nontargeted methods for adulteration detection. In: Appendix XVIII. 2016. Rockville, USA:US pharmacopei.p. 1510.

30. Available at: https://www.accessdata.fda.gov/cdrh_docs/reviews/DEN170019.pdf.

31. Available at: https://www.accessdata.fda.gov/cdrh_docs/reviews/K190266.pdf.

32. Seger C, Salzmann L. After another decade: LC-MS/MS became routine in clinical diagnostics. Clin Biochem 2020;82:2–11.

33. Available at: https://www.fda.gov/files/drugs/published/Bioanalytical-Method-Validation-Guidance-for-Industry.pdf.

34. Eberlin LS, Margulis K, Planell-Mendez I, et al. Pancreatic cancer surgical resection margins: molecular assessment by mass spectrometry imaging. PLoS Med 2016;13(8):e1002108.

35. Eberlin LS, Tibshirani RJ, Zhang J, et al. Molecular assessment of surgical-resection margins of gastric cancer by mass-spectrometric imaging. Proc Natl Acad Sci U S A 2014;111(7):2436–41.

36. Santoro AL, Drummond RD, Silva IT, et al. In situ DESI-MSI lipidomic profiles of breast cancer molecular subtypes and precursor lesions. Cancer Res 2020; 80(6):1246–57.

37. Zhang J, Li SQ, Lin JQ, et al. Mass spectrometry imaging enables discrimination of renal oncocytoma from renal cell cancer subtypes and normal kidney tissues. Cancer Res 2020;80(4):689–98.

38. Woolman M, Ferry I, Kuzan-Fischer CM, et al. Rapid determination of medulloblastoma subgroup affiliation with mass spectrometry using a handheld picosecond infrared laser desorption probe. Chem Sci 2017;8(9):6508–19.

39. Katz L, Woolman M, Talbot F, et al. Dual laser and desorption electrospray ionization mass spectrometry imaging using the same interface. Anal Chem 2020; 92(9):6349–57.

40. Banerjee S, Wong AC, Yan X, et al. Early detection of unilateral ureteral obstruction by desorption electrospray ionization mass spectrometry. Sci Rep 2019;9(1): 11007.

41. Banerjee S, Zare RN, Tibshirani RJ, et al. Diagnosis of prostate cancer by desorption electrospray ionization mass spectrometric imaging of small metabolites and lipids. Proc Natl Acad Sci U S A 2017;114(13):3334–9.

42. Eberlin LS, Gabay M, Fan AC, et al. Alteration of the lipid profile in lymphomas induced by MYC overexpression. Proc Natl Acad Sci U S A 2014;111(29): 10450–5.

43. Margulis K, Chiou AS, Aasi SZ, et al. Distinguishing malignant from benign microscopic skin lesions using desorption electrospray ionization mass spectrometry imaging. Proc Natl Acad Sci U S A 2018;115(25):6347–52.

44. Sans M, Gharpure K, Tibshirani R, et al. Metabolic markers and statistical prediction of serous ovarian cancer aggressiveness by ambient ionization mass spectrometry imaging. Cancer Res 2017;77(11):2903–13.

45. Vijayalakshmi K, Shankar V, Bain RM, et al. Identification of diagnostic metabolic signatures in clear cell renal cell carcinoma using mass spectrometry imaging. Int J Cancer 2020;147(1):256–65.

46. Bodai Z, Cameron S, Bolt F, et al. Effect of electrode geometry on the classification performance of rapid evaporative ionization mass spectrometric (REIMS) bacterial identification. J Am Soc Mass Spectrom 2018;29(1):26–33.

47. Esslinger S, Riedl J, Fauhl-Hassek C. Potential and limitations of non-targeted fingerprinting for authentication of food in official control. Food Res Int 2014;60: 189–204.

48. Cavanna D, Righetti L, Elliott C, et al. The scientific challenges in moving from targeted to non-targeted mass spectrometric methods for food fraud analysis: a proposed validation workflow to bring about a harmonized approach. Trends Food Sci Technology 2018;80:223–41.

49. McGrath TF, Haughey SA, Patterson J, et al. What are the scientific challenges in moving from targeted to non-targeted methods for food fraud testing and how can they be addressed? – spectroscopy case study. Trends Food Sci Technology 2018;76:38–55.

50. Silva AAR, Cardoso MR, Rezende LM, et al. Multiplatform investigation of plasma and tissue lipid signatures of breast cancer using mass spectrometry tools. Int J Mol Sci 2020;21(10):3611.

51. Barry JA, Ait-Belkacem R, Hardesty WM, et al. Multicenter validation study of quantitative imaging mass spectrometry. Anal Chem 2019;91(9):6266–74.

52. Porcari AM, Zhang J, Garza KY, et al. Multicenter study using desorption-electrospray-ionization-mass-spectrometry imaging for breast-cancer diagnosis. Anal Chem 2018;90(19):11324–32.

53. Kreidler SM, Muller KE, Grunwald GK, et al. GLIMMPSE: online power computation for linear models with and without a baseline covariate. J Stat Softw 2013; 54(10):i10.

54. Blaise BJ. Data-driven sample size determination for metabolic phenotyping studies. Anal Chem 2013;85(19):8943–50.

55. Blaise BJ, Correia G, Tin A, et al. Power analysis and sample size determination in metabolic phenotyping. Anal Chem 2016;88(10):5179–88.

56. Martin JC, Maillot M, Mazerolles G, et al. Can we trust untargeted metabolomics? Results of the metabo-ring initiative, a large-scale, multi-instrument interlaboratory study. Metabolomics 2015;11(4):807–21.

57. Smilde AK, Jansen JJ, Hoefsloot HCJ, et al. ANOVA-simultaneous component analysis (ASCA): a new tool for analyzing designed metabolomics data. Bioinformatics 2005;21(13):3043–8.

58. Franceschi P, Vrhovsek U, Mattivi F, et al. Metabolic biomarker identification with few samples. Chemometrics in Practical Applications. London, UK: IntechOpen Limited; 2012.

59. Xia J, Broadhurst DI, Wilson M, et al. Translational biomarker discovery in clinical metabolomics: an introductory tutorial. Metabolomics 2013;9(2):280–99.

60. Sumner LW, Amberg A, Barrett D, et al. Proposed minimum reporting standards for chemical analysis. Metabolomics 2007;3(3):211–21.

61. Schymanski EL, Jeon J, Gulde R, et al. Identifying small molecules via high resolution mass spectrometry: communicating confidence. Environ Sci Technol 2014;48(4):2097–8.

62. Pettus BJ, Chalfant CE, Hannun YA. Ceramide in apoptosis: an overview and current perspectives. Biochim Biophys Acta 2002;1585(2–3):114–25.

63. Roszkowska A, Yu M, Bessonneau V, et al. Tissue storage affects lipidome profiling in comparison to in vivo microsampling approach. Sci Rep 2018;8(1): 6980.

64. Thomas RL Jr, Matsko CM, Lotze MT, et al. Mass spectrometric identification of increased C16 ceramide levels during apoptosis. J Biol Chem 1999;274(43): 30580–8.

65. Eberlin LS, Ferreira CR, Dill AL, et al. Nondestructive, histologically compatible tissue imaging by desorption electrospray ionization mass spectrometry. Chembiochem 2011;12(14):2129–32.

66. Brochu F, Plante PL, Drouin A, et al. Mass spectra alignment using virtual lockmasses. Sci Rep 2019;9(1):8469.

67. Eikel D, Vavrek M, Smith S, et al. Liquid extraction surface analysis mass spectrometry (LESA-MS) as a novel profiling tool for drug distribution and metabolism analysis: the terfenadine example. Rapid Commun Mass Spectrom 2011;25(23):3587–96.

68. Annesley TM. Ion suppression in mass spectrometry. Clin Chem 2003;49(7): 1041–4.

69. Eberlin LS, Norton I, Orringer D, et al. Ambient mass spectrometry for the intraoperative molecular diagnosis of human brain tumors. Proc Natl Acad Sci U S A 2013;110(5):1611–6.

70. Correa DN, Santos JM, Eberlin LS, et al. Forensic chemistry and ambient mass spectrometry: a perfect couple destined for a happy marriage? Anal Chem 2016;88(5):2515–26.

71. Ifa DR, Jackson AU, Paglia G, et al. Forensic applications of ambient ionization mass spectrometry. Anal Bioanal Chem 2009;394(8):1995–2008.

72. Rigano F, Mangraviti D, Stead S, et al. Rapid evaporative ionization mass spectrometry coupled with an electrosurgical knife for the rapid identification of Mediterranean Sea species. Anal Bioanal Chem 2019;411(25):6603–14.

73. Verplanken K, Stead S, Jandova R, et al. Rapid evaporative ionization mass spectrometry for high-throughput screening in food analysis: the case of boar taint. Talanta 2017;169:30–6.

74. van der Kwast TH, Lopes C, Santonja C, et al. Guidelines for processing and reporting of prostatic needle biopsies. J Clin Pathol 2003;56(5):336–40.

75. Howell LP, Gandour-Edwards R, Folkins K, et al. Adequacy evaluation of fine-needle aspiration biopsy in the breast health clinic setting. Cancer 2004; 102(5):295–301.

76. Taylor MD, Northcott PA, Korshunov A, et al. Molecular subgroups of medulloblastoma: the current consensus. Acta Neuropathol 2012;123(4):465–72.

77. Kool M, Korshunov A, Remke M, et al. Molecular subgroups of medulloblastoma: an international meta-analysis of transcriptome, genetic aberrations, and clinical data of WNT, SHH, Group 3, and Group 4 medulloblastomas. Acta Neuropathol 2012;123(4):473–84.

78. Gottardo NG, Hansford JR, McGlade JP, et al. Medulloblastoma down under 2013: a report from the third annual meeting of the international medulloblastoma working group. Acta Neuropathol 2014;127(2):189–201.

79. Porter NA, Caldwell SE, Mills KA. Mechanisms of free radical oxidation of unsaturated lipids. Lipids 1995;30(4):277–90.

80. Green DR, Galluzzi L, Kroemer G. Cell biology. Metabolic control of cell death. Science 2014;345(6203):1250256.
81. Brown HA, Marnett LJ. Introduction to lipid biochemistry, metabolism, and signaling. Chem Rev 2011;111(10):5817–20.
82. Ahnoff M, Cazares LH, Skold K. Thermal inactivation of enzymes and pathogens in biosamples for MS analysis. Bioanalysis 2015;7(15):1885–99.
83. Woolman M, Tata A, Bluemke E, et al. An assessment of the utility of tissue smears in rapid cancer profiling with desorption electrospray ionization mass spectrometry (DESI-MS). J Am Soc Mass Spectrom 2017;28(1):145–53.
84. Fatou B, Saudemont P, Leblanc E, et al. In vivo real-time mass spectrometry for guided surgery application. Sci Rep 2016;6:25919.

Glycan Imaging Mass Spectrometry

Progress in Developing Clinical Diagnostic Assays for Tissues, Biofluids, and Cells

Calvin R.K. Blaschke, BS, Colin T. McDowell, BS,
Alyson P. Black, BS, Anand S. Mehta, DPhil, Peggi M. Angel, PhD,
Richard R. Drake, PhD*

KEYWORDS

- Imaging mass spectrometry • Glycosylation • Biomarkers • Clinical diagnostics

KEY POINTS

- Imaging mass spectrometry (IMS) is a powerful tool to link changes in disease-associated N-linked glycosylation with histopathology features in standard formalin-fixed paraffin-embedded tissue samples.
- N-glycan IMS has revealed specific carbohydrate structures and motifs associated with a variety of cancers with the potential for development into clinical biomarkers.
- Advancements in instrumentation and sample preparation can effectively address N-glycan IMS limitations, such as sialic acid stability, structural isomer determination, and matrix effects.
- The tissue N-glycan IMS workflow has been adapted to clinical biofluids, cultured cells, and immunoarray-captured glycoproteins for detection of changes in glycosylation associated with disease.

INTRODUCTION

Protein glycosylation is a highly prevalent posttranslational modification involving the attachment of oligosaccharides, most commonly to a serine/threonine residue (O-linked glycosylation) or an asparagine residue (N-linked glycosylation). Glycosylation is a highly regulated process with more than 300 enzymes involved in their biosynthesis and processing in a non–template-driven manner. This process is done by a series of sequential reactions involving a wide array of glycotransferases that attach

C.R K. Blaschke and C.T. McDowell contributed equally to the work.
Department of Cell and Molecular Pharmacology, Medical University of South Carolina, 173 Ashley Avenue, BSB 358, Charleston, SC 29425, USA
* Corresponding author.
E-mail address: draker@musc.edu

single monosaccharides from nucleotide sugar donors, as well as different glycosidases that remove individual monosaccharides.[1] The expression, activity, and localization of these enzymes are sensitive to the physiologic state of the cell. Estimated to occur on more than half of human proteins,[2] N-linked glycosylation has essential roles in protein folding, molecular trafficking, signal transduction, cell-cell interactions, and many other processes.[3–6] Glycans serve as one of the initial points of contact during cell-to-cell interactions, so therefore disease changes in glycan biosynthesis can be more apparent than disease-related changes associated with gene mutations and proteins.[7] Alterations in N-linked glycosylation have been found in a variety of diseases, including but not limited to cancer,[8] inflammatory arthritis,[9] liver fibrosis/cirrhosis,[10] schizophrenia,[11] type 2 diabetes,[12] ischemic stroke,[13] and Parkinson disease.[14] Particularly for cancers, most US Food and Drug Administration–approved cancer biomarkers comprise circulating glycoproteins or carbohydrate antigens for measurement in blood.[7,8,15–18] Glycoproteins can be ideal biomarkers because they enter circulation from tissues or blood cells through active secretion or leakage, making them assessable for analysis through serum. These current biomarker targets (eg, prostate-specific antigen or the carbohydrate antigen CA19-9) are far from ideal and have many limitations because of specificity and other factors.[17]

There are many analytical approaches that have been applied to the analysis of disease-associated changes in the glycan constituents of glycoproteins in tissues biofluids. Reviews highlighting some of these methods are as follows, and include use of carbohydrate-binding lectins,[19,20] anti–carbohydrate antigen antibodies,[21] glycan microarrays,[22] high-performance liquid chromatography (HPLC), and mass spectrometry (MS).[23–27] Historically, there have been persistent challenges across all glycan analysis methods related to generally poor affinities of antibodies for carbohydrate epitopes, weak and nonspecific binding affinities of lectins, distinguishing isomeric species, and issues of extensive sample processing for HPLC and MS. The aforementioned reviews highlight progress in these areas, and the field in general is moving toward development of potential clinical and diagnostic assay workflows. Our group has recently developed several glycan targeted assays using imaging MS (IMS) approaches,[28–33] including extensive detailed protocols.[34,35] Originally developed for spatial analysis of N-glycans in tissues,[28–30] different adaptations of the approach have been developed for analysis of N-glycans of biofluids,[31] cells,[32] and captured proteins[33] directly on glass slides. These approaches are distinguished by their overall throughput, ease and speed of preparation, and robustness. Using mass spectrometers equipped with matrix-assisted laser desorption/ionization (MALDI) sources for these assays, the consistent and reproducible detection of N-glycan structures in clinical samples has the potential to mature into clinical assays analogous to the MALDI MS–based assays that have transformed clinical microbiology identification of bacterial and other pathogen species.[36,37] The workflows, strengths, limitations, and clinical implications of using MALDI-IMS N-glycan analysis are discussed with examples for the analysis of tissues, clinical biofluids, cultured cells, and immunoarray-captured glycoproteins.

METHOD OVERVIEW AND APPLICATIONS OF N-GLYCAN MATRIX-ASSISTED LASER DESORPTION/IONIZATION IMAGING MASS SPECTROMETRY OF TISSUES

MALDI-IMS analysis of proteins in tissues was initially described in 1997 by the Caprioli laboratory,[38] and the field has rapidly evolved to facilitate the spatial distribution and identification of all classes of biomolecules using multiple types of mass spectrometers and ionization sources.[39–41] Key to the success of MALDI-IMS in identification of disease-specific biomolecules has been the ability to correlate IMS data with histopathologic classification of tissue subtypes by standard histology and immunohistochemistry stains.[42,43] Specific application of N-glycan–targeted MALDI-IMS was reported initially in fresh frozen tissues in 2013, followed a year later in formalin-fixed paraffin-embedded (FFPE) tissue sections.[28–30] The method workflow is summarized in **Fig. 1**. The key to the approach is to spray a molecular coating of peptide N-glycosidase F (PNGase F) on the tissue, an enzyme that cleaves the N-linked glycan structures at their site of attachment to an asparagine residue on the glycoprotein carrier. The released N-glycans are detected in the mass spectrometer after application of an organic acid matrix and ionization by laser desorption, using a rastered grid of locations generally 40 to 100 μm apart across the entire tissue. A two-dimensional distribution map of the peak intensities of each released glycan is generated by analysis of the cumulative spectra obtained from each spot on the tissue. Use of a solvent sprayer has allowed robust and reproducible sample preparatory workflows to evolve that facilitate large-scale analysis of clinical tissue cohorts.[28,44] This basic workflow has been used by multiple laboratories to characterize the N-glycan distributions for multiple cancer types, including breast,[45–47] prostate,[48,49] liver,[48,50] pancreas,[29,51] ovary,[52] colon,[30,53] sarcoma,[54,55] kidney,[43] and lung,[56] as well as in cardiac[57,58] and other tissue types.[43,45,46,50,57,59,60] An example MALDI-IMS N-glycan image of a human colorectal adenocarcinoma tissue is shown in **Fig. 2**. This example clearly shows the histopathologic colocalization of specific glycans to different regions of the tissue, including tumor and adjacent normal crypt, stroma, and smooth muscle regions. The overlay and single glycan images shown are representative of more than 100 distinct glycan species that can be detected in this tissue.

Based on thousands of analyses of individual FFPE tumor tissue slides and tumor cores in tissue microarray slides, several advantages to N-glycan MALDI-IMS are evident relative to other MALDI-IMS targets. A major advantage with regard to clinical

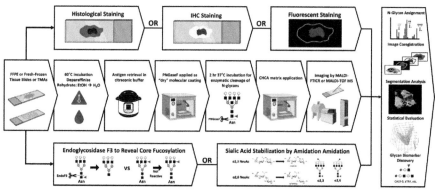

Fig. 1. Overview of MALDI-IMS workflow and orthogonal analyses. (*Middle row*) A standardized N-glycan IMS workflow including dewaxing and rehydration, antigen retrieval, release of N-glycans by peptide N-glycosidase F (PNGase F), matrix application, and imaging by MALDI-MS. (*Bottom row*) Endoglycosidase F3 and sialic acid-amidation adaptations to the N-glycan IMS workflow for detection of fucosylation and sialylation isomers, respectively. (*Top row*) Orthogonal imaging techniques, including histologic, immunohistochemistry, and immunofluorescence staining. (*Panel, right side*) Integration of data from traditional, adapted, and orthogonal analyses for comprehensive characterization of the tissue N-glycome. CHCA, α-Cyano-4-hydroxycinnamic acid; FTICR, Fourier-ransform Ion Cyclotron Resonance; TMA, tissue microarray; TOF, time of flight.

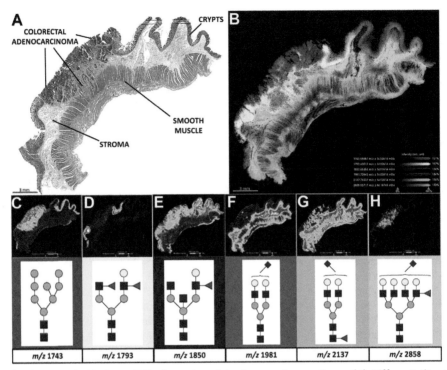

Fig. 2. Example N-glycan IMS of a colorectal adenocarcinoma tissue. (*A*) Different tissue structures (hematoxylin-eosin). (*B*) Overlay image of 6 N-glycan structures that colocalize with distinct tissue regions. (*C–H*) Individual N-glycan heatmaps from overlay in panel B Hex8HexNAc2 (*red*), Hex4HexNAc4Fuc2 (*yellow*), Hex4HexNAc5Fuc1 (*purple*), Hex5HexNAc4α2,6NeuAc1 (*blue*), Hex5HexNAc4Fuc1α2,3NeuAc1 (*green*), and Hex7HexNAc6Fuc1α2,6-NeuAc1 (*orange*). Monosaccharide unit symbols: mannose (*green circle*), galactose (*yellow circle*), N-acetylglucosamine (*blue square*), fucose (*red triangle*), α2,3-linked sialic acid (*purple diamond, right shifted*), α2,6-linked sialic acid (*purple diamond, left shifted*).

translation is the ability to perform these analyses on FFPE tissues, thereby leveraging the predominant specimen type found in clinical histopathology laboratories and tissue biorepositories. The MALDI-IMS workflow fits seamlessly into the pathology laboratory, because it uses the same tissue sections required for pathologic evaluation without additional patient interactions. Similarly, the processing steps for the method before PNGase F application are essentially the same as standard histology practices for tissue staining and immunohistochemistry (see **Fig. 1**). Because the N-glycans lack free amine groups and are thus not cross-linked by formalin, it has been shown that only dewaxing, but not antigen retrieval, can be used effectively to obtain glycan signals.[54,61] For analytical considerations using the basic workflow, the released glycans are detected directly from the tissue without need of enrichment or derivatization. The glycans detected depend entirely on the activity of the PNGase F, thus any background signal caused by tissue is minimal. The use of the automated solvent sprayer to apply a reproducible thin molecular coating of PNGase F ensures minimal diffusion and excellent colocalization of glycans to their sites of origin.[34] In addition, because of the sequential nature of their biosynthesis, the basic structural compositions of the N-glycans that can arise are known and well documented.[3,30] For MALDI-IMS, this results in highly reproducible detection of a core number of ∼ 40 N-glycan species in normal and tumor tissues that can be used for basic biostatistical comparisons across conditions. These glycans also serve as the scaffolds for disease-associated increases in sialic acid and fucose modifications resulting from expression of different genes in the fucosyltransferase and sialyltransferase families. Some tumor types also are characterized by increases in glycans with bisecting N-acetylglucosamine structures and poly-lactosamine extensions.[46,62] Thus, in cancer tissues, such as that shown in **Fig. 2**, the numbers of N-glycans detected generally increase in proportion to pathology grade and tumor stage. The masses of these added sugars are also well defined; therefore, determinations of the structural compositions of these larger N-glycans are straightforward. This type of data is essentially a glycan bar code that can be applied to clinical cohorts for biostatistical analysis and biomarker studies, described in more detail later.

LIMITATIONS AND METHOD ADAPTATIONS FOR N-GLYCAN MATRIX-ASSISTED LASER DESORPTION/IONIZATION IMAGING MASS SPECTROMETRY

There are several limitations of N-glycan IMS that are inherent to the properties of N-glycans, as well as instrumentation and method limitations that are related to the use of MALDI as the ionization source. These limitations include differentiating structural isomers, stability of sialic acid glycans to MALDI ionization, suppression of N-glycan signal because of matrix effects, the detection of glycans with masses greater than $m/z = 4000$, and decreased sensitivity with increased spatial resolution. Strategies used to overcome these limitations, along with other potential approaches, are summarized as follows.

There are many structural isomers that can arise from the sequential addition of sugars in N-glycans. Notably, there are 13 fucosyltransferase genes that encode a family of enzymes responsible for the addition of fucose to N-glycan structures. Outer arm fucose residues (ie, those attached to sugars on the branched antennae) are primarily attached via either α-1,2 (FUT1,2) or α-1,3 and α-1,4 (FUT3,4,6,7,9-11) linkages. Core fucosylation at the terminal N-acetylglucosamine residue attached to the Asn of the protein is done exclusively by FUT8, with an α-1,6 linkage.[63] For sialic acids, 2 main glycosyltransferases, ST3Gal1 and ST6Gal1, from a gene family of more than 15 sialyltransferases, are responsible for the addition of α-2,3 or α-2,6 linked sialic acids to the terminal galactose moieties on branched N-glycans.[64] The presence or absence of these different fucose and sialic acid linkages largely depends on the specific gene expression patterns in each tissue and cell type, as well as disease state, thus each tissue analyzed by MALDI-IMS has many possible glycans that could be present. Distinguishing these structural isomers has always been a challenge for MS analysis of N-glycans, and especially for MALDI-MS approaches. Although accurate masses and glycan compositions can be readily determined, the specific antennae location and anomeric linkages associated with fucose and sialic acid modifications are difficult to establish. Recently, several enzymatic and chemical adaptations to the standard workflow have been developed to solve some of the difficulties associated with detection of fucosylation and sialylation isomers (see **Fig. 1**). The distinction between core or terminal fucosylation is important to determine, because increases in core fucosylation are associated with more aggressive cancer phenotypes and poorer patient outcomes.[50,65–67] Recently, a new enzyme has been incorporated into the N-glycan MALDI-IMS workflow. Termed endoglycosidase F3 (Endo F3), this enzyme specifically cleaves N-glycans with core fucose residues, between the 2 N-acetylglucosamine residues on the N-glycan chitobiose core in the presence of a core fucose residue (see **Fig. 1**). This process results in a mass shift of 349 mass unit. to the released N-glycan, representing the loss of 1 N-acetylglucosamine and 1 fucose.[48] N-glycans lacking a core fucose are poor substrates for this enzyme. Subsequently, incorporation of this enzyme into N-glycan IMS strategies resolves core versus outer arm fucosylation isomers.[48] Using Endo F3 and PNGase F in a 1:10 ratio can free both core and terminally fucosylated N-glycan isomers in a single tissue analysis. Distinguishing the isomeric linkages of α-2,3 versus α-2,6 sialic acid residues on N-glycans is further complicated by the lability of sialic acid residues during MALDI ionization, as well as by the fact that the negative charge of sialic acids typically forms salt adducts with additional sodium ions, reducing sensitivity of detection.[68,69] To overcome these challenges, an on-tissue chemical amidation approach has been developed that stabilizes sialic acid residues before preparation for MALDI-IMS.[53] Critically, in addition to stabilization, this method differentially derivatizes α-2,3 and α-2,6 linked sialic acid N-glycans with stable amide and dimethylamide groups, respectively. This disparate incorporation induces a distinct mass shift in sialylated N-glycans that allows the specific detection of α-2,3 versus α-2,6 isomers in IMS-derived data. Examples of these anomeric differences are also shown in the data for the colorectal tumor in **Fig. 2**.

Common to all types of MALDI-MS and MALDI-IMS is the blunting of analyte signal caused by interference by the chemical matrix. The laser desorption process and subsequent transfer of analytes into the gas phase fragments the matrix and results in the ejection of matrix ions into the mass spectrometer alongside N-glycan ions. These additional m/z peaks detected complicate the analysis of MALDI-generated mass spectra and may lead to overall signal suppression and potential obfuscation of N-glycan peaks, especially those of lower molecular weight or lower intensities. These challenges are currently being overcome by several approaches. Simplest among them is the incorporation of ammonium salts (acetate, formate, or phosphate),[70,71] either as a matrix solution component or as a postmatrix application spray, into the MALDI-IMS workflow.[70] Ammonium salts help prevent the formation of matrix adducts, thereby breaking up the larger matrix crystal clusters that differentially absorb laser energy and lead to signal suppression.[72–74] Recently, a strategy to reduce matrix interference specific to N-glycan MALDI-MS has been developed. The use of a modified reactive DHB (DHBH) in combination with catalytic DHB allows the simultaneous derivatization of cleaved N-glycans and cocrystallization of these analytes with this novel matrix mixture.[75] Subsequently, this workflow modification has shown utility not only in the reduction of matrix interference but also in the boosting of N-glycan signal and the quantification of these species.

Mammalian N-glycans are known to range in molecular weight from m/z 933 (the common Hex3HexNAc2 N-glycan core) to more than 10,000 m/z for very large polylactosamine-containing structures. The analysis of such higher-molecular-weight N-glycan structures is typically difficult via traditional MALDI-IMS workflows, which, even when optimized for increased signal from the upper m/z range, struggle to reliably detect masses greater than 5000 m/z. Here again, multiple strategies are available to address this shortcoming. Chemical derivatization of tissue homogenate followed by MALDI time-of-flight (TOF) detection and N-glycan identification via a matched filtering algorithm analysis recently allowed the identification of polylactosamine N-glycan ions up to ~14,000 m/z.[76] Also, a novel instrumentation approach may soon be able to overcome this obstacle. Laser positronization-coupled MALDI-IMS (MALDI-2) uses a secondary laser source to further ionize the analyte plume ejected by the primary laser.[77] In doing so, low abundance and hard-to-detect ions receive a signal boost and are therefore detected more robustly. Because this second laser ionizes the analyte cloud as a whole, it has the potential to increase signal across the entire mass range. The aforementioned methods to address glycan isomer determinations begin to unravel some of the major glycan isomer challenges, but not all. There remain other challenges associated with distinguishing modifications such as terminal N-acetylglucosamine residues versus bisecting N-acetylglucosamine, as well as determining which antennae branch is modified. The recent introduction of trapped ion mobility separated TOF MS instruments into the MALDI-IMS space helps to deconvolute this complexity.[78,79] Structural isomers from an ion packet of the same *m/z* migrate through an electric field in a manner proportional to their structural geometry, allowing high resolving power and very fine discrimination of structures that are compositionally the same but differ in their precise linkages. This technology has already shown utility in parsing out N-glycan isomers.[80]

Although the breadth of detectable molecular information in IMS can identify many analytes, the routine image resolution obtained at the tissue and cell levels is at the 20-μm level and higher. Other imaging modalities, such as fluorescent microscopy and super-resolution microscopy,[81] as well as alternative IMS methods such as TOF-SIMS and MIBI-TOF,[41,82–84] allow imaging of analytes at submicrometer resolution. This level of resolution is not currently achievable using standard MALDI-IMS. Advances in MALDI-IMS platforms, such as transmission geometry MALDI-IMS, and associated methodologies have progressively increased spatial resolution, but at the cost of signal intensity.[85] To achieve cellular or subcellular resolutions in IMS, the typically large laser pixel size (~25 μm) must be reduced. In doing so, the amount of laser energy directed at the tissue in a single shot necessarily decreases, resulting in the detection of fewer analytes and an overall reduction in signal strength.[83] This trade-off is potentially addressed by MALDI-2, which can compensate for this loss of molecular information through increasing signal after desorption, and has shown a pixel size as low as 600 nm.[86] It is yet to be determined whether single-micrometer resolution capabilities are necessary to improve current N-glycan MALDI-IMS data, particularly in the context of clinical assay development.

EMERGING USES OF N-GLYCAN MATRIX-ASSISTED LASER DESORPTION/IONIZATION IMAGING MASS SPECTROMETRY FOR CANCER TISSUE BIOMARKERS AND DIAGNOSTICS

In our group, the use of tissue microarrays (TMAs) representing liver, kidney, pancreas, and breast cancers in conjunction with whole tissue slices have allowed larger cohorts of samples to be analyzed.[29,36,51,59] The resulting glycan peak lists can be combined with clinical patient data, pathology information, and genetic subtyping information to evaluate detection of glycan changes as potential diagnostic biomarkers. For breast cancer, an initial study evaluated TMAs representing Her2+ and triple-negative breast cancer (TNBC) subtypes.[46] There were minor differences in glycan metabolism, with Her2+ tumors having higher levels of triantennary and tetra-antennary precursors relative to TNBC, whereas TNBC tumors had higher levels of high-mannose N-glycans. A more striking finding was the detection of N-glycans with poly-lactosamine extensions in the most aggressive tumor cores of Her2+ and TNBC, as well as in a cohort of metastatic and primary tumor tissue pairs. The ability to detect these poly-lactosamine N-glycans in the most advanced breast tumors was further evaluated in a tissue microarray of 145 breast tumor cores, primarily representing intraductal ductal carcinomas, with outcome and survival data.[47] Analysis of the resulting N-glycan peak lists indicated that the presence of core-fucosylated tetra-antennary N-glycan with a single N-acetyllactosamine extension indicated tissues associated with poor outcome, including lymph node metastasis, recurrent disease, and reduced survival. The presence of core fucose was confirmed using EndoF3. The authors hypothesize that this approach could be applied to diagnostic biopsy and/or primary resection tissues to improve identification of women with more lethal forms of breast cancer.

Another example is the use of N-glycans detected in TMAs from hepatocellular carcinoma (HCC) tissue to predict survival outcomes. From an N-glycan imaging analysis of 138 tumor cores and whole tissues, there were 10 N-glycans at levels identified as significantly increased relative to normal or cirrhotic liver tissues. These tumor glycans primarily had increased levels of fucosylation. There was also a distinct subset of tumors with a primary tetra-antennary branched glycan as the main difference. In 1 subset, a nonfucosylated structure (Hex7HexNAc6) predominated, and the other subset had monofucosylated and difucosylated versions (Hex7-HexNAc6Fuc1/2). The tumors associated with the fucosylated glycans had poorer outcomes and decreased survival times relative to the samples with the nonfucosylated glycan. A follow-up study using EndoF3 digestion of the same TMAs further indicated that, for the monofucosylated and difucosylated glycans, those that were core fucosylated had worse survival times than those without.[48] The demonstration that core-fucosylated N-glycans in HCC tissues are associated with poorer outcomes is consistent with many previous studies reporting overall increases in core fucosylation for HCC.[50,59,66,67,87–90] Current efforts are focused on applying the same N-glycan MALDI-IMS workflows to a large cohort of genetically subtyped HCC tumors (S1, S2, S3) that are correlated with clinical parameters such as tumor size, extent of cellular differentiation, serum alpha fetoprotein levels, signaling pathways, treatment responses, and outcomes.[91,92] Similar strategies are ongoing to link established cancer biomarkers and other clinical correlates with N-glycans from prostate and pancreatic cancer tissue cohorts, including three-dimensional (3D) strategies and linkage for prostate with clinical MRI coregistrations.[49]

N-GLYCAN IMAGING MASS SPECTROMETRY OF CLINICAL BIOFLUIDS

Blood-based samples are attractive mediums for biomarker detection because of the availability of large clinical cohorts, as well as the cost-effective and minimally invasive manner of collection. Although there have been several MALDI-MS strategies developed for analysis of N-glycan profiles in biofluids, there are a limited number of high-throughput methodologies capable of analyzing the current-day clinical cohorts that commonly contain thousands of samples. One of the largest plasma N-glycan studies analyzed more than 2144 individuals by MALDI-MS to identify associations of plasma N-glycans with markers of inflammation and metabolic health.[93] The MALDI-MS workflow involved the release of N-glycans with PNGase F, sialic acid stabilization by ethyl esterification, purification by hydrophilic interaction liquid chromatography (HILIC), incorporation of chemical matrix, and spotting onto a MALDI target plate, with many of the steps completed with an automated liquid-handling robot.[94] This workflow would be further optimized by limiting derivatization side-reactions, decreasing batch-to-batch variances by changing the HILIC stationary phase, and using MALDI-FTICR instead of MALDI-TOF.[95] A nonautomated form of this workflow was adapted for dried blood spot N-glycan analysis, which represents an even less invasive collection strategy.[96] These strategies have been used to investigate a wide array of diseases, including multiple myeloma,[97] inflammatory bowel disease,[98] rheumatoid arthritis,[24] and colorectal cancer.[99] These extensive studies on large sample cohorts have established N-glycan detection in plasma by MALDI-IMS as a clinically relevant assay for clinical diagnostic laboratories.

Another method for serum N-glycan analysis uses an enrichment strategy termed glycoblotting, in which beads conjugated with hydrazide groups bind N-glycans released from serum samples.[100] Not only are the bead-bound N-glycans purified with a series of washes but the sialic acids are stabilized by methyl esterification. The hydrazide groups with attached N-glycans are released from the bead by reduction with dithiothreitol. The enriched N-glycans are spotted directly onto a MALDI target plate, mixed with matrix, and analyzed by MALDI-TOF MS. The processing time of this workflow was reduced when combined with an automated sample-processing system that can perform most of the steps.[101] Glycoblotting-based serum analysis has been used extensively to find many disease-specific N-glycan alterations.[102–107] The clinical utility of this workflow is distinguished by the minimal hands-on time.

Recently, Blaschke and colleagues[31] developed a rapid high-throughput IMS workflow for serum and plasma N-glycan profiling. In this workflow, serum or plasma is spotted on an amine-reactive hydrogel-coated slide resulting in the covalent binding of proteins to the slide during a 1-hour incubation in a humidity chamber. It is well known that lipids and salts suppress the N-glycan signal during IMS. Accordingly, samples are delipidated with washes of Carnoy solution (60% ethanol, 30% chloroform, 10% glacial acetic acid), and desalted with a water wash. The rest of the workflow follows the tissue processing steps shown in **Fig. 1**. The slide is sprayed with PNGase F, incubated for 2 hours, and sprayed with matrix. The sample-processing time is significantly decreased by avoiding lengthy derivatization and purification steps typically found in clinical biofluid N-glycan profiling methods. A slide with 28 samples can be processed and imaged in less than 11 hours on an FTICR instrument. Multiple slides can be processed together to increase throughput with minimal additional time requirements, and other MS instruments can be used for quicker MS data acquisition. This workflow can detect 75 N-glycans from less than 1 μL of serum or plasma. The simplicity, speed, and sensitivity of this method make it highly amenable for use as a clinical assay.

Shown in **Fig. 3** are example data for detection of 6 N-glycans detected from the serum of a patient with liver cirrhosis and a patient with HCC. Alterations in the glycosylation of glycoproteins found in tissue and serum during the development of HCC have been well documented.[87,90,108,109] For example, increased fucosylation of biantennary, triantennary, and tetra-antennary glycans have been found in several studies.[50,59,66,67,87–90] Consistent with this, fucosylated biantennary N-glycans were detected at higher levels in the HCC sample relative to the cirrhotic sample. Analysis of larger clinical patient sample cohorts is ongoing, as well as strategies for automated sample spotting and processing.

N-GLYCAN IMAGING MASS SPECTROMETRY OF CULTURED CELLS

Although liquid chromatography coupled to MS (LC-MS) is the most common technique for analyzing the N-glycan profile of cells,[110,111] Angel and colleagues[32] used MALDI-IMS to create an alternative method that is rapid and robust. In this novel method, cells are cultured on a conventional cell culture chamber slide array, fixated with neutral buffered formalin, and delipidated with Carnoy solution. Subsequent steps mirror the tissue imaging workflow, except for a few minor alterations. Compared with tissue, this cell imaging method had the greatest sensitivity by applying less PNGase F and matrix. In addition, ammonium phosphate monobasic was sprayed onto the slide after the matrix application to minimize the formation of signal-suppressing matrix clusters. Signal detected from N-glycans in the serum-

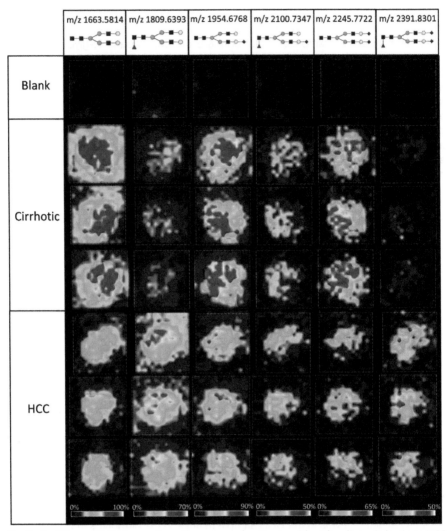

Fig. 3. Profiling of 6 N-glycans from the serum of patients with either liver cirrhosis or HCC using the method described by Blaschke and colleagues.[31] Monosaccharide unit symbols are as indicated in **Fig. 2**.

containing media was found to be highly reproducible and could be subtracted out as background. The arrays can be normalized for cellular protein levels by incorporating a traditional protein-binding stain, Coomassie G-250, after MS data acquisition. With this simple workflow, 88 cell chambers can be N-glycan profiled within 1 day, including overnight MS analysis, with minimal hands-on time. This ability represents a vast improvement compared with the lengthy sample-processing steps needed when using LC-MS.

Using this method, Angel and colleagues[32] were able to reproducibly detect 70 N-glycoforms from a variety of human and mouse cell lines. The N-glycan profiles contained a variety of N-glycan structures, including high mannose and fucose and sialic acid containing biantennary, triantennary, and tetra-antennary N-glycans. As discussed, N-glycans have important roles in cell signaling and require precise regulation. With no additional processing time, N-glycan turnover could be detected by integrating an isotopic detection of amino sugars with a glutamine labeling approach (**Fig. 4**). The incorporation of ^{15}N amide glutamine into all N-acetylglucosamine, N-acetylgalactosamine, and sialic acids creates a distinct mass shift in all newly synthesized N-glycans. As shown in **Fig. 4** at near-single-cell resolution, turnover rates of individual N-glycans can be determined by comparing the intensities of the unlabeled and labeled forms over several time points. The rapid and robust array-based MALDI-IMS approach is an innovative solution to the analytical challenge of glycomic studies in cultured cells and serves as a foundational launching point for basic, translational, and pharmaceutical investigations into mechanisms of N-glycan function and regulation in cultured cells.

N-GLYCAN IMAGING MASS SPECTROMETRY OF IMMUNOARRAY-CAPTURED GLYCOPROTEINS

Recently developed immunoassays modified for glycosylation analysis of isolated glycoproteins have the potential for robust analysis of large cohorts of clinical samples. Disease-associated alterations in the glycosylation of immunoglobulin G (IgG),[112] α1-acid glycoprotein (AGP),[113] haptoglobin,[114] transferrin,[115] and alpha -fetoprotein[108] have been shown and could have utility as biomarkers. There have been several methods for high-throughput N-glycan analysis of immunocaptured glycoproteins using lectin microarrays to identify carbohydrate structural motifs.[116,117] Essentially, these techniques work like the common ELISA (enzyme-linked immunosorbent assay)

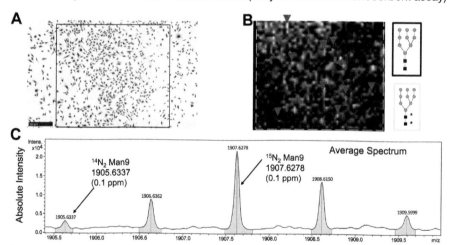

Fig. 4. N-glycan turnover in cell culture by imaging MS strategies. Human aortic endothelial cells are grown in ^{15}N glutamine for 48 hours, adding an ^{15}N at every N-acetylglucosamine, N-acetylgalactose, and N-acetylneuraminic acid. Fully labeled N-glycans with complete incorporation of ^{15}N indicate a complete turnover of that N-glycan. (*A*) Human aortic endothelial cells are grown with ^{15}N glutamine on a conventional cell chamber slide. This image shows cells that have been stained after IMS analysis with Coomassie blue to allow normalization to cell numbers and protein content. (*B*) Example image data of the same region of cultured cells. Image is of high-mannose N-glycan Man9. Cells were scanned at a step size of 25 μm. Blue indicates no turnover, yellow indicates full turnover, white is partial incorporation of the label, indicating a slower turnover rate for some cells (*red arrows*). (*C*) Example N-glycan profile showing the high-mannose peak Man9. Monosaccharide unit symbols are as indicated in **Fig. 2**.

technique where the protein of interest is captured by an antibody and analyzed with multiple lectins. Although the large number of different lectins can cover a wide range of glycan structures, the low binding affinities and undefined specificities of most lectins limit their utility for analysis of clinical cohorts. In addition, lectins are unable to determine the entire composition or type of the bound glycan.

These limitations can be mitigated by an MS-based approach. Darebna and colleagues[118] developed a method for detecting altered glycoforms of transferrin that are characteristic of heavy alcohol abuse using MALDI-IMS. The workflow includes electrospraying antitransferrin antibody onto an indium tin oxide glass slide, capturing transferrin from serum, washing the slide, and applying matrix. The glycoforms of transferrin have distinct masses that can be detected by MALDI-TOF MS. The peak intensities of the glycoforms were compared between healthy and alcoholic patient serum samples. This immunoassay approach avoids the previously discussed limitations of lectin microarrays and the lengthy sample cleanup necessary for traditional protein glycosylation techniques.

Black and colleagues[33,35] expanded and adapted the immunoarray approach for glycoprotein analysis with the development of antibody panel–based (APB) N-glycan imaging. In this novel technique, antibodies are spotted onto a microscope slide in an array, glycoproteins are specifically captured from patient biofluids, and N-glycans are enzymatically released for analysis by MALDI-IMS. The multiplexing of antibodies can be used to analyze the intensities of hundreds of glycans from hundreds of glycoproteins from 1 μL of serum in a single imaging run. This method only requires 8 hours of hands-on time and has the possibility of being automated with a liquid-handling robot. To ensure N-glycan changes are not caused by varying protein levels, a saturating amount of protein must be added to the antibody array. This technique relies on the binding affinity and specificity of the antibodies and requires validation of each antibody used. **Fig. 5** shows representative APB N-glycan imaging data obtained from serum analysis of 7 glycoproteins simultaneously. APB N-glycan imaging improves

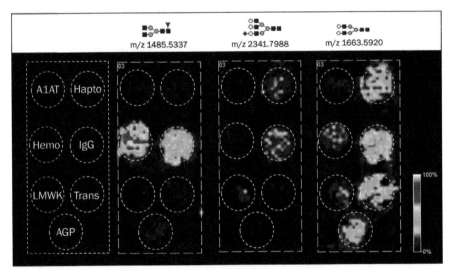

Fig. 5. Antibody panel based imaging of 3 N-glycans for 7 glycoproteins captured from a pool of serum collected from patients with liver cirrhosis using the method described by Black and colleagues.[33] Monosaccharide unit symbols are as indicated in **Fig. 2**. A1AT, alpha-1-antitrypsin; AGP, alpha-1-acid glycoprotein; Hapto, haptoglobin; Hemo, hemoglobin; IgG, immunoglobulin G; LMWK, low-molecular-weight kininogen; Trans, transferrin.

the sensitivity and simplicity of glycoprotein analysis in a manner suitable for robust analysis of large clinical cohorts.

FUTURE DIRECTIONS

For each of the indicated applications, multiple steps in the workflow can be optimized to move toward clinical assay implementation. Glycan profiling of biopsy tissues in particular, such as those frequently obtained for liver, prostate, and breast cancer assessments, or kidney for diabetes, could be integrated with current pathology practices. A recent report described a rapid MALDI-IMS analysis workflow for frozen tissues that required only ~ 5 total minutes of preparation and analysis time integrated into a pathology laboratory setting.[119] It is unlikely that this timeline could be adapted directly to N-glycan IMS workflows, because the PNGase F digestion step is required, but it is feasible to incorporate components of the method optimization strategies that were reported. The optimized tissue imaging workflows are also applicable to multimodal IMS combinations with other glycosidases and proteases, as well as large-scale 3D imaging.[49,120,121] A recent study illustrates how coregistering IMS data with data from MRI of prostate cancer allows 3D reconstruction of tumors and tumor margins and spatial identification of specific oncometabolites.[120] Other enzymes can also readily be incorporated into the workflow. As described for incorporating Endo F3 into the current workflows, other enzymes targeting different glycoconjugates could also be used. For example, another endoglycosidase, endoglycosidase S (Endo S), cleaves N-glycans in a similar manner to Endo F3 but is specific to N-glycans present on human immunoglobulin G91. This enzyme could find applicability in each of the tissue, biofluid, and antibody microarray workflows. In addition, the slide-based biofluid assays described for antibody capture arrays and total serum and plasma glycan analysis and immunoarrays could be adapted to other types of biofluid targets. A major new target is the adaptation of these approaches to characterizing the N-glycan constituents of immune cell subsets, either using peripheral blood mononuclear cell isolates or from flow cytometry sorted fractions. Different components of the antibody capture array, amine-reactive slide, and cell culturing strategies are being applied to clinical immune cell isolates. This area remains largely unexplored for N-glycans but could lead to major diagnostic advances for cancer immunotherapy and infectious disease monitoring.

SUMMARY

This article provides an overview of the clinically relevant applications of this rapidly evolving glycan MALDI-IMS methodology and highlights its potential value as a clinical diagnostic tool. Applying N-glycan MALDI-IMS workflows to the study of tissues, cells, and biofluids has expanded the ability to link glycobiology to mechanisms of disease and improved biomarker detection capabilities. The development and integration of technological advancements in mass spectrometers and sample preparation techniques have expanded, and will continue to expand, the use of MALDI-IMS for the robust analysis of clinical specimens.

ACKNOWLEDGMENTS

This research was supported in part by the South Carolina Smart State Centers of Economic Excellence (R.R. Drake, A.S. Mehta) and National Institutes of Health grants U01CA242096 (R.R. Drake, A.S. Mehta, P.M. Angel); R41DK124058 (A.S. Mehta), U01CA226052 (A.S. Mehta, R.R. Drake), Biorepository and Tissue Analysis Shared

Resource, Hollings Cancer Center, Medical University of South Carolina (P30 CA138313), and T32GM132055 to C.T. McDowell.

DISCLOSURE

R.R. Drake, P.M. Angel, and A.S. Mehta disclose partial ownership interests in 2 companies: GlycoPath, LLC, Mt Pleasant, South Carolina, and N-Zyme Scientifics, Doylestown, Pennsylvania.

REFERENCES

1. Nairn AV, York WS, Harris K, et al. Regulation of glycan structures in animal tissues: transcript profiling of glycan-related genes. J Biol Chem 2008;283(25): 17298–313.
2. Apweiler R, Hermjakob H, Sharon N. On the frequency of protein glycosylation, as deduced from analysis of the SWISS-PROT database. Biochim Biophys Acta 1999;1473(1):4–8.
3. Moremen KW, Tiemeyer M, Nairn AV. Vertebrate protein glycosylation: diversity, synthesis and function. Nat Rev Mol Cell Biol 2012;13(7):448–62.
4. Tanaka T, Yoneyama T, Noro D, et al. Aberrant N-glycosylation profile of serum immunoglobulins is a diagnostic biomarker of urothelial carcinomas. Int J Mol Sci 2017;18(12):1–14.
5. Gu J, Isaji T, Xu Q, et al. Potential roles of N-glycosylation in cell adhesion. Glycoconj J 2012;29(8–9):599–607.
6. Shental-Bechor D, Levy Y. Folding of glycoproteins: toward understanding the biophysics of the glycosylation code. Curr Opin Struct Biol 2009;19(5):524–33.
7. Kailemia MJ, Park D, Lebrilla CB. Glycans and glycoproteins as specific biomarkers for cancer. Anal Bioanal Chem 2017;409(2):395–410.
8. Adamczyk B, Tharmalingam T, Rudd PM. Glycans as cancer biomarkers. Biochim Biophys Acta 2012;1820(9):1347–53.
9. Albrecht S, Unwin L, Muniyappa M, et al. Glycosylation as a marker for inflammatory arthritis. Cancer Biomarkers 2014;14:17–28.
10. Blomme B, Van Steenkiste C, Callewaert N, et al. Alteration of protein glycosylation in liver diseases. J Hepatol 2009;50(3):592–603.
11. Williams SE, Mealer RG, Scolnick EM, et al. Aberrant glycosylation in schizophrenia: a review of 25 years of post-mortem brain studies. Mol Psychiatry 2020. https://doi.org/10.1038/s41380-020-0761-1.
12. Lemmers RFH, Vilaj M, Urda D, et al. IgG glycan patterns are associated with type 2 diabetes in independent European populations. Biochim Biophys Acta 2017;1861(9):2240–9.
13. Liu D, Zhao Z, Wang A, et al. Ischemic stroke is associated with the pro-inflammatory potential of N-glycosylated immunoglobulin G. J Neuroinflammation 2018;15(1):123.
14. Russell AC, Šimurina M, Garcia MT, et al. The N-glycosylation of immunoglobulin G as a novel biomarker of Parkinson's disease. Glycobiology 2017;27(5): 501–10.
15. Barton JG, Bois JP, Sarr MG, et al. Predictive and prognostic value of CA 19-9 in resected pancreatic adenocarcinoma. J Gastrointest Surg 2009;13(11):2050–8.
16. Drake RR. Glycosylation and cancer: moving glycomics to the forefront. Adv Cancer Res 2015;126:1–10.
17. Ludwig JA, Weinstein JN. Biomarkers in cancer staging, prognosis and treatment selection. Nat Rev Cancer 2005;5(11):845–56.

18. Song E, Mechref Y. Defining glycoprotein cancer biomarkers by MS in conjunction with glycoprotein enrichment. Biomark Med 2015;9(9):835–44.
19. Brooks SA. Lectin histochemistry: Historical perspectives, state of the art, and the future. Methods Mol Biol 2017;1560:93–107.
20. Cummings RD. The repertoire of glycan determinants in the human glycome. Mol Biosyst 2009;5(10):1087–104.
21. Sterner E, Flanagan N, Gildersleeve JC. Perspectives on anti-glycan antibodies gleaned from development of a community Resource database. ACS Chem Biol 2016;11(7):1773–83.
22. Smith DF, Cummings RD. Application of microarrays for deciphering the structure and function of the human glycome. Mol Cell Proteomics 2013;12(4):902–12.
23. Ruhaak LR, Xu G, Li Q, et al. Mass spectrometry approaches to glycomic and glycoproteomic analyses. Chem Rev 2018;118(17):7886–930.
24. Reiding KR, Bondt A, Hennig R, et al. High-throughput Serum N-glycomics: method comparison and application to study rheumatoid arthritis and pregnancy-associated changes. Mol Cell Proteomics 2019;18(1):3–15.
25. Gray C, Flitsch SL. Methods for the high resolution analysis of glycoconjugates. In: Witczak ZJ, Bielsk R, editors. Coupling and decoupling of diverse molecular units in glycosciences. Cham, Switzerland: Springer International Publishing; 2017. p. 225–67. https://doi.org/10.1007/978-3-319-65587-1_11.
26. Reider B, Jarvas G, Krenkova J, et al. Separation based characterization methods for the N-glycosylation analysis of prostate-specific antigen. J Pharm Biomed Anal 2021;194:113797.
27. Zhang L, Luo S, Zhang B. Glycan analysis of therapeutic glycoproteins Glycan analysis of therapeutic glycoproteins. MAbs 2016;8(2):205–15.
28. Powers TW, Jones EE, Betesh LR, et al. Matrix assisted laser desorption ionization imaging mass spectrometry workflow for spatial profiling analysis of N-linked Glycan expression in tissues. Anal Chem 2013;85(20):9799–806.
29. Powers TW, Neely BA, Shao Y, et al. MALDI imaging mass spectrometry profiling of N-glycans in formalin-fixed paraffin embedded clinical tissue blocks and tissue microarrays. PLoS One 2014;9(9):1–11.
30. Drake RR, Powers TW, Jones EE, et al. MALDI mass spectrometry imaging of N-linked glycans in cancer tissues. Adv Cancer Res 2017;134:85–116.
31. Blaschke C, Black A, Mehta AS, et al. Rapid N-glycan profiling of serum and plasma by a novel slide based imaging mass spectrometry workflow. J Am Soc Mass Spectrom 2020. https://doi.org/10.1021/jasms.0c00213.
32. Angel PM, Saunders J, Clift CL, et al. A rapid array-based approach to N-glycan profiling of cultured cells. J Proteome Res 2019;18(10):3630–9.
33. Black AP, Liang H, West CA, et al. A novel mass spectrometry platform for multiplexed N-glycoprotein biomarker discovery from patient biofluids by antibody panel based N-glycan imaging. Anal Chem 2019;91(13):8429–35.
34. Drake RR, Powers TW, Norris-Caneda K, et al. In situ imaging of N-glycans by MALDI imaging mass spectrometry of fresh or formalin-fixed paraffin-embedded tissue. Curr Protoc Protein Sci 2018;94(1):1–21.
35. Black AP, Angel PM, Drake RR, et al. Antibody panel based N-glycan imaging for N-glycoprotein biomarker discovery. Curr Protoc Protein Sci 2019;98(1). https://doi.org/10.1002/cpps.99.
36. Drake RR, Boggs SR, Drake SK. Pathogen identification using mass spectrometry in the clinical microbiology laboratory. J Mass Spectrom 2011;46(12):1223–32.

37. Kostrzewa M. Application of the MALDI Biotyper to clinical microbiology: progress and potential. Expert Rev Proteomics 2018;15(3):193–202.

38. Caprioli RM, Farmer TB, Gile J. Molecular imaging of Biological samples: localization of peptides and proteins using MALDI-TOF MS. Anal Chem 1997;69(23): 4751–60.

39. Schwamborn K, Caprioli RM. Molecular imaging by mass spectrometry-looking beyond classical histology. Nat Rev Cancer 2010;10(9):639–46.

40. Angel PM, Caprioli RM. Matrix-assisted laser desorption ionization imaging mass spectrometry: in situ molecular mapping. Biochemistry 2013;52(22): 3818–28.

41. Porta Siegel T, Hamm G, Bunch J, et al. Mass spectrometry imaging and integration with other imaging modalities for greater molecular understanding of Biological tissues. Mol Imaging Biol 2018;20(6):888–901.

42. Deutskens F, Yang J, Caprioli RM. High spatial resolution imaging mass spectrometry and classical histology on a single tissue section. J Mass Spectrom 2011;46(6):568–71.

43. Drake RR, McDowell C, West C, et al. Defining the human kidney N-glycome in normal and cancer tissues using MALDI imaging mass spectrometry. J Mass Spectrom 2020;55(4):e4490.

44. Gemperline E, Rawson S, Li L. Optimization and comparison of multiple MALDI matrix application methods for small molecule mass spectrometric imaging. Anal Chem 2014;86(20):10030–5.

45. Scott DA, Norris-Caneda K, Spruill L, et al. Specific N-linked glycosylation patterns in areas of necrosis in tumor tissues. Int J Mass Spectrom 2019;437:69–76.

46. Scott DA, Casadonte R, Cardinali B, et al. Increases in tumor N-glycan polylactosamines associated with advanced HER2-positive and triple-negative breast cancer tissues. PROTEOMICS – Clin Appl 2019;13(1):1800014.

47. Herrera H, Dilday T, Uber A, et al. Core-Fucosylated Tetra-Antennary N-Glycan Containing A Single N-acetyllactosamine branch is associated with poor survival outcome in breast cancer. Int J Mol Sci 2019;20(10):2528.

48. West CA, Liang H, Drake RR, et al. A new enzymatic approach to distinguish fucosylation isomers of N-linked glycans in tissues using MALDI imaging mass spectrometry. J Proteome Res 2020. https://doi.org/10.1021/acs.jproteome.0c00024.

49. Drake RR, Angel PM, Wu J, et al. How else can we approach prostate cancer biomarker discovery? Expert Rev Mol Diagn 2020;20(2):123–5.

50. West CA, Wang M, Herrera H, et al. N-linked glycan branching and fucosylation are increased directly in Hcc tissue as determined through in situ glycan imaging. J Proteome Res 2018;17(10):3454–62.

51. McDowell CT, Klamer Z, Hall J, et al. Imaging mass spectrometry and lectin analysis of N-linked glycans in carbohydrate antigen defined pancreatic cancer tissues. Mol Cell Proteomics 2021;20. https://doi.org/10.1074/mcp.ra120.002256.

52. Briggs MT, Condina MR, Ho YY, et al. MALDI mass spectrometry imaging of early- and late-stage serous ovarian cancer tissue reveals stage-specific N- glycans. Proteomics 2019;19(21–22):1800482.

53. Holst S, Heijs B, De Haan N, et al. Linkage-specific in situ sialic acid derivatization for N-glycan mass spectrometry imaging of formalin-fixed paraffin-embedded tissues. Anal Chem 2016;88(11):5904–13.

54. Heijs B, Holst S, Briaire-De Bruijn IH, et al. Multimodal mass spectrometry imaging of N-glycans and proteins from the same tissue section. Anal Chem 2016; 88(15):7745–53.
55. Heijs B, Holst-Bernal S, de Graaff MA, et al. Molecular signatures of tumor progression in myxoid liposarcoma identified by N-glycan mass spectrometry imaging. Lab Investig 2020;100(9):1252–61.
56. Carter CL, Parker GA, Hankey KG, et al. MALDI-MSI spatially maps N-glycan alterations to histologically distinct pulmonary pathologies following irradiation. Sci Rep 2020;10(1):1–14.
57. Angel PM, Baldwin HS, Gottlieb Sen D, et al. Advances in MALDI imaging mass spectrometry of proteins in cardiac tissue, including the heart valve. Biochim Biophys Acta 2017;1865(7):927–35.
58. Angel PM, Drake RR, Park Y, et al. Spatial N-glycomics of the human aortic valve in development and pediatric endstage congenital aortic valve stenosis. J Mol Cell Cardiol 2021;154:6–20.
59. Powers T, Holst S, Wuhrer M, et al. Two-dimensional N-glycan distribution mapping of hepatocellular carcinoma tissues by MALDI-imaging mass spectrometry. Biomolecules 2015;5(4):2554–72.
60. Briggs MT, Kuliwaba JS, Muratovic D, et al. MALDI mass spectrometry imaging of N-glycans on tibial cartilage and subchondral bone proteins in knee osteoarthritis. Proteomics 2016;16(11–12):1736–41.
61. Ostasiewicz P, Zielinska DF, Mann M, et al. Proteome, phosphoproteome, and N-glycoproteome are quantitatively preserved in formalin-fixed paraffin-embedded tissue and analyzable by high-resolution mass spectrometry. J Proteome Res 2010;9(7):3688–700.
62. Porterfield M, Zhao P, Han H, et al. Discrimination between adenocarcinoma and normal pancreatic ductal fluid by proteomic and glycomic analysis. J Proteome Res 2014;13(2):395–407.
63. Schneider M, Al-Shareffi E, Haltiwanger RS. Biological functions of fucose in mammals. Glycobiology 2017;7(27):601–18.
64. Harduin-Lepers A, Vallejo-Ruiz V, Krzewinski-Recchi MA, et al. The human sialyltransferase family. Biochimie 2001;83(8):727–37.
65. Keeley TS, Yang S, Lau E. The diverse contributions of fucose linkages in cancer. Cancers (Basel) 2019;11(9). https://doi.org/10.3390/cancers11091241.
66. Comunale MA, Rodemich-Betesh L, Hafner J, et al. Linkage specific fucosylation of alpha-1-antitrypsin in liver cirrhosis and cancer patients: implications for a biomarker of hepatocellular carcinoma. PLoS One 2010;5(8):e12419.
67. Comunale MA, Wang M, Hafner J, et al. Identification and development of fucosylated glycoproteins as biomarkers of primary hepatocellular carçinoma. J Proteome Res 2009;8(2):595–602.
68. Nie H, Li Y, Sun XL. Recent advances in sialic acid-focused glycomics. J Proteomics 2012;75(11):3098–112.
69. Reiding KR, Blank D, Kuijper DM, et al. High-throughput profiling of protein N-Glycosylation by MALDI-TOF-MS employing linkage-specific sialic acid esterification. Anal Chem 2014. https://doi.org/10.1021/ac500335t.
70. Ucal Y, Ozpinar A. Improved spectra for MALDI MSI of peptides using ammonium phosphate monobasic in MALDI matrix. J Mass Spectrom 2018;53(8): 635–48.
71. Angel PM, Spraggins JM, Baldwin HS, et al. Enhanced sensitivity for high spatial resolution lipid analysis by negative ion mode matrix assisted laser desorption ionization imaging mass spectrometry. Anal Chem 2012;84(3):1557–64.

72. Zhu X, Papayannopoulos IA. Improvement in the detection of low concentration protein digests on a MALDI TOF/TOF Workstation by reducing-cyano-4-hydroxycinnamic acid adduct ions. Vol 14. The association of biomolecular Resource Facilities; 2003. Available at: http://pmc/articles/PMC2279961/?report=abstract. Accessed August 18, 2020.

73. Smirnov IP, Zhu X, Taylor T, et al. Suppression of α-cyano-4-hydroxycinnamic acid matrix clusters and reduction of chemical noise in MALDI-TOF mass spectrometry. Anal Chem 2004;76(10):2958–65.

74. Asara JM, Allison J. Enhanced detection of phosphopeptides in matrix-assisted laser desorption/ionization mass spectrometry using ammonium salts. J Am Soc Mass Spectrom 1999;10(1):35–44.

75. Zhao X, Guo C, Huang Y, et al. Combination strategy of reactive and catalytic matrices for qualitative and quantitative profiling of N-glycans in MALDI-MS. Anal Chem 2019. https://doi.org/10.1021/acs.analchem.9b02144.

76. Bern M, Brito AE, Pang PC, et al. Polylactosaminoglycan glycomics: Enhancing the detection of high-molecular-weight N-glycans in matrix-assisted laser desorption ionization time-of-flight profiles by matched filtering. Mol Cell Proteomics 2013;12(4):996–1004.

77. Barré FPY, Paine MRL, Flinders B, et al. Enhanced sensitivity using maldi imaging coupled with laser postionization (maldi-2) for pharmaceutical research. Anal Chem 2019;91(16):10840–8.

78. Fernandez-Lima F. Trapped Ion Mobility Spectrometry: past, present and future trends. Int J Ion Mobil Spectrom 2016;19(2–3):65–7.

79. Spraggins JM, Djambazova KV, Rivera ES, et al. High-performance molecular imaging with MALDI Trapped Ion-Mobility Time-of-Flight (timsTOF) mass spectrometry. Anal Chem 2019;91(22):14552–60.

80. Pu Y, Ridgeway ME, Glaskin RS, et al. Separation and identification of isomeric glycans by selected accumulation-trapped ion mobility spectrometry-electron activated dissociation tandem mass spectrometry. Anal Chem 2016;88(7):3440–3.

81. Sigal YM, Zhou R, Zhuang X. Visualizing and discovering cellular structures with super-resolution microscopy. Science 2018;361(6405):880–7.

82. Keren L, Bosse M, Thompson S, et al. MIBI-TOF: a multiplexed imaging platform relates cellular phenotypes and tissue structure. Sci Adv 2019;5(10):eaax5851.

83. Ščupáková K, Balluff B, Tressler C, et al. Cellular resolution in clinical MALDI mass spectrometry imaging: the latest advancements and current challenges. Clin Chem Lab Med 2020;58(6):914–29.

84. Keren L, Bosse M, Marquez D, et al. A structured tumor-immune microenvironment in triple negative breast cancer revealed by multiplexed ion Beam imaging. Cell 2018;174(6):1373–87.e19.

85. Zavalin A, Todd EM, Rawhouser PD, et al. Direct imaging of single cells and tissue at sub-cellular spatial resolution using transmission geometry MALDI MS. J Mass Spectrom 2012;47(11):i.

86. Niehaus M, Soltwisch J, Belov ME, et al. Transmission-mode MALDI-2 mass spectrometry imaging of cells and tissues at subcellular resolution. Nat Methods 2019;16(9):925–31.

87. Block TM, Comunale MA, Lowman M, et al. Use of targeted glycoproteomics to identify serum glycoproteins that correlate with liver cancer in woodchucks and humans. Proc Natl Acad Sci U S A 2005;102(3):779–84.

88. Wang M, Sanda M, Comunale MA, et al. Changes in the glycosylation of kininogen and the development of a kininogen-based algorithm for the early detection of HCC. Cancer Epidemiol Biomarkers Prev 2017;26(5):795–803.
89. Wang M, Long RE, Comunale MA, et al. Novel fucosylated biomarkers for the early detection of hepatocellular carcinoma. Cancer Epidemiol Biomarkers Prev 2009;18(6):1914–21.
90. Comunale MA, Lowman M, Long RE, et al. Proteomic analysis of serum associated fucosylated glycoproteins in the development of primary hepatocellular carcinoma. J Proteome Res 2006;5(2):308–15.
91. Hoshida Y, Nijman SMB, Kobayashi M, et al. Integrative transcriptome analysis reveals common molecular subclasses of human hepatocellular carcinoma. Cancer Res 2009. https://doi.org/10.1158/0008-5472.CAN-09-1089.
92. Tan PS, Nakagawa S, Goossens N, et al. Clinicopathological indices to predict hepatocellular carcinoma molecular classification. Liver Int 2016;36(1):108–18.
93. Reiding KR, Ruhaak LR, Uh H-W, et al. Human Plasma N-glycosylation as analyzed by matrix-assisted laser desorption/ionization-fourier transform ion cyclotron resonance-MS associates with markers of inflammation and metabolic health*. Mol Cell Proteomics 2017;16(2):228–42.
94. Bladergroen MR, Reiding KR, Hipgrave Ederveen AL, et al. Automation of high-throughput mass spectrometry-based plasma n-glycome analysis with linkage-specific sialic acid esterification. J Proteome Res 2015;14(9):4080–6.
95. Vreeker GCM, Nicolardi S, Bladergroen MR, et al. Automated plasma glycomics with linkage-specific sialic acid esterification and ultrahigh resolution MS. Anal Chem 2018. https://doi.org/10.1021/acs.analchem.8b02391.
96. Vreeker GCM, Bladergroen MR, Nicolardi S, et al. Dried blood spot N-glycome analysis by MALDI mass spectrometry. Talanta 2019;205:120104.
97. Zhang Z, Westhrin M, Bondt A, et al. Serum protein N-glycosylation changes in multiple myeloma. Biochim Biophys Acta 2019;1863(5):960–70.
98. Clerc F, Novokmet M, Dotz V, et al. Plasma N-glycan signatures are associated with features of inflammatory bowel diseases. Gastroenterology 2018;155(3):829–43.
99. de Vroome SW, Holst S, Girondo MR, et al. Serum N-glycome alterations in colorectal cancer associate with survival. Oncotarget 2018;9(55):30610–23.
100. Miura Y, Hato M, Shinohara Y, et al. BlotGlycoABC™, an integrated glycoblotting technique for rapid and large scale clinical glycomics. Mol Cell Proteomics 2008;7(2):370–7.
101. Nishimura SI. Toward automated glycan analysis. Adv Carbohydr Chem Biochem 2011;65:219–71.
102. Miyahara K, Nouso K, Saito S, et al. Serum glycan markers for evaluation of disease activity and prediction of clinical course in patients with ulcerative colitis. PLoS One 2013;8(10):e74861.
103. Gebrehiwot AG, Melka DS, Kassaye YM, et al. Exploring serum and immunoglobulin G N-glycome as diagnostic biomarkers for early detection of breast cancer in Ethiopian women. BMC Cancer 2019;19(1):588.
104. Hatakeyama S, Amano M, Tobisawa Y, et al. Serum N-glycan alteration associated with Renal cell carcinoma detected by high throughput glycan analysis. J Urol 2014;191(3):805–13.
105. Gizaw ST, Ohashi T, Tanaka M, et al. Glycoblotting method allows for rapid and efficient glycome profiling of human Alzheimer's disease brain, serum and cerebrospinal fluid towards potential biomarker discovery. Biochim Biophys Acta 2016;1860(8):1716–27.

106. Matsumoto T, Hatakeyama S, Yoneyama T, et al. Serum N-glycan profiling is a potential biomarker for castration-resistant prostate cancer. Sci Rep 2019;9(1):16761.

107. Noro D, Yoneyama T, Hatakeyama S, et al. Serum aberrant N-glycan profile as a marker associated with early antibody-mediated rejection in patients receiving a living donor kidney transplant. Int J Mol Sci 2017;18(8). https://doi.org/10.3390/ijms18081731.

108. Johnson PJ, Poon TCW, Hjelm NM, et al. Structures of disease-specific serum alpha-fetoprotein isoforms. Br J Cancer 2000;83(10):1330–7.

109. Mehta A, Herrera H, Block T. Glycosylation and liver cancer. Adv Cancer Res 2015;126:257–79.

110. Shajahan A, Heiss C, Ishihara M, et al. Glycomic and glycoproteomic analysis of glycoproteins—a tutorial. Anal Bioanal Chem 2017;409(19):4483–505.

111. Domann PJ, Pardos-Pardos AC, Fernandes DL, et al. Separation-based glycoprofiling approaches using fluorescent labels. Proteomics 2007;7(S1):70–6.

112. Vilaj M, Gudelj I, Trbojević-Akmačić I, Lauc G, Pezer M. IgG Glycans as a Biomarker of Biological Age. In: Moskalev A, editor. Biomarkers of Human Aging. Healthy Ageing and Longevity, vol 10. Springer, Cham; 2019. p. 81–99. Available at: https://link.springer.com/chapter/10.1007%2F978-3-030-24970-0_7.

113. Imre T, Kremmer T, Héberger K, et al. Mass spectrometric and linear discriminant analysis of N-glycans of human serum alpha-1-acid glycoprotein in cancer patients and healthy individuals. J Proteomics 2008;71(2):186–97.

114. Tsai H-Y, Boonyapranai K, Sriyam S, et al. Glycoproteomics analysis to identify a glycoform on haptoglobin associated with lung cancer. Proteomics 2011;11(11):2162–70.

115. Bones J, Mittermayr S, O'Donoghue N, et al. Ultra performance liquid chromatographic profiling of serum N-glycans for fast and efficient identification of cancer associated alterations in glycosylation. Anal Chem 2010;82(24):10208–15.

116. Hirabayashi J. Concept, strategy and realization of lectin-based glycan profiling. J Biochem 2008;144(2):139–47.

117. Chen S, LaRoche T, Hamelinck D, et al. Multiplexed analysis of glycan variation on native proteins captured by antibody microarrays. Nat Methods 2007;4(5):437–44.

118. Darebna P, Spicka J, Kucera R, et al. Detection and quantification of carbohydrate-deficient transferrin by MALDI-compatible protein chips prepared by Ambient ion soft landing. Clin Chem 2018;64(9):1319–26.

119. Basu SS, Regan MS, Randall EC, et al. Rapid MALDI mass spectrometry imaging for surgical pathology. Npj Precis Oncol 2019;3(1). https://doi.org/10.1038/s41698-019-0089-y.

120. Abdelmoula WM, Regan MS, Lopez BGC, et al. Automatic 3D nonlinear registration of mass spectrometry imaging and magnetic resonance imaging data. Anal Chem 2019;91(9):6206–16.

121. Clift CL, Mehta AS, Drake RR, et al. Multiplexed imaging mass spectrometry of the extracellular matrix using serial enzyme digests from formalin-fixed paraffin-embedded tissue sections. Anal Bioanal Chem 2020;1–11. https://doi.org/10.1007/s00216-020-03047-z.

Matrix-Assisted Laser Desorption Ionization Time-of-Flight for Fungal Identification

Anna F. Lau, PhD, D(ABMM)

KEYWORDS

- MALDI-TOF MS • Mold • Yeast • Rapid identification • Review

KEY POINTS

- MALDI-TOF MS has demonstrated excellent performance for rapid yeast identification. Updated databases provide accurate identification of cryptic species that have increased resistance to antifungal agents.
- MALDI-TOF MS for mold identification is highly reliant on the use of in-house developed databases to supplement the manufacturer's databases.
- Successful implementation of MALDI-TOF MS for mold identification has been demonstrated; however, culture methods, extraction methods, databases, and acquisition methods lack standardization.
- Early research shows that MALDI-TOF MS may be used to detect antifungal resistance in yeasts; poor performance was demonstrated for mold.

INTRODUCTION

The identification of yeasts and filamentous fungi (molds) has historically relied on a combination of phenotypic and morphologic characteristics. Recent studies, however, have uncovered a vast array of species-complexes and cryptic species that can only be reliably identified by the use of more delineated and targeted testing platforms, such as sequencing and matrix-assisted laser desorption ionization time-of-flight mass spectrometry (MALDI-TOF MS). Around 2010, MALDI-TOF MS technology was launched into the clinical microbiology field, and was a game-changer because clinical laboratories could now identify organisms from crude protein suspensions within minutes, at low processing costs, and minimal processing time. The accuracy of MALDI-TOF MS for organism identification was equivalent to DNA sequencing, and its ease of use led it to be a highly sought after platform in multiple fields including clinical microbiology, veterinary care, the food and beverage industry, and environmental microbiology. Currently, there are two main MALDI-TOF MS systems on the market:

Sterility Testing Service, Department of Laboratory Medicine, Clinical Center, National Institutes of Health, 10 Center Drive, Room 2C306, Bethesda, MD 20892, USA
E-mail address: anna.lau@nih.gov

Clin Lab Med 41 (2021) 267–283
https://doi.org/10.1016/j.cll.2021.03.006
0272-2712/21/Published by Elsevier Inc.

labmed.theclinics.com

MALDI BioTyper (MBT; Bruker Scientific, Billerica, MA) and VITEK MS (BioMerieux, Marcy-l'Etoile, France). The MBT was cleared by the Food and Drug Administration (FDA) in 2013 for bacteria and yeast identification only, although a separate FilFungal database became available in 2012 for mold identification for research use only (RUO). In contrast, the VITEK MS version 3.0 was cleared by the FDA in 2017 with a database that expanded bacteria, yeasts, mold, and mycobacteria. The critical role of databases and processing methods is addressed in this review because methods have evolved considerably over time.

Today, MALDI-TOF MS has become a mainstream platform in most clinical laboratories for bacterial identification. However, its application in clinical mycology for yeast and mold identification has been lagging, which is mostly attributable to the lack of standardized processes and poor fungal database representation. In fact, clinical mycology expertise is sorely lacking in laboratories worldwide and MALDI-TOF MS has the potential to fill this knowledge gap. In 2018, a survey of 348 tertiary care hospitals in China were reported to have insufficient clinical mycology testing capacity.[1] Similarly, 241 laboratories surveyed across seven Asian countries reported that only 53.5% of participants had designated mycology laboratories and that nearly all participants used traditional microscopy and culture methods for fungal identification; only 16.9% and 12.3% performed DNA sequencing and MALDI-TOF MS, respectively, for organism identification.[2] Participant surveys from the 2019 and 2020 College of American Pathologists mycology proficiency testing program, which comprises up to approximately 1000 laboratories (most from the United States), also showed that only approximately 50% of laboratories used MALDI-TOF MS for yeast identification, whereas less than 7% of laboratories used MALDI-TOF MS for mold identification.

Clearly, the waning availability of mycologic expertise in front-line laboratories and the need for accurate fungal identification (particularly for capture of cryptic species that generally have higher resistance profiles) leads to an urgent need to expand the application of MALDI-TOF MS into clinical mycology. This review provides an overview of the current status of MALDI-TOF MS for fungal identification, including key findings in the literature, processing and database considerations, updates in technology, and future prospects.

MATRIX-ASSISTED LASER DESORPTION IONIZATION TIME-OF-FLIGHT MASS SPECTROMETRY FOR YEAST IDENTIFICATION

Researchers have reported excellent performance of Bruker MBT and VITEK MS platforms for yeast identification, although success rates can vary considerably depending on the organism challenge set, database version, extraction processing method, and acceptable cutoff threshold. Thus, data from the literature must be interpreted with caution. For yeast identification, high reproducibility has been reported across different testing environments, instruments, operators, reagent and target slide lots, and sample positioning patterns through multicenter studies.[3,4] The advantages of MALDI-TOF MS for yeast identification compared with phenotypic platforms is overwhelmingly evident. **Table 1** highlights some of the common misidentifications by traditional phenotypic methods that are resolved by the use of MALDI-TOF MS. Many discrepancies involve delineations within the species complexes, such as *Candida glabrata* complex (*C glabrata*, *Candida nivariensis*, *Candida bracarensis*) and *Candida parapsilosis* complex (*C parapsilosis*, *Candida metapsilosis*, *Candida orthopsilosis*). A study of 182 yeast isolates demonstrated a 91% concordance between the MBT and the API 20C AUX biochemical panel; discordant results were attributed to rarely encountered and phenotypically difficult to identify organisms.[5]

Table 1
Common misidentifications associated with traditional identification platforms that are resolved by MALDI-TOF MS

Accurate Identification (Method)	Misidentification (Traditional Method)	Reference
Candida albicans (MBT)	Candida famata (VITEK 2)	Garza-Gonzalez et al,[8] 2020; Chao et al,[9] 2014
Candida auris (MBT)	Candida catenulata (Microscan), C famata (Microscan), Candida haemulonii (VITEK 2), Candida inconspicua (Microscan)	Ceballos-Garzon et al,[6] 2019
Candida dubliniensis (MBT)	C albicans (Microscan, Phoenix Yeast ID)	Ceballos-Garzon et al,[6] 2019; Chao et al,[9] 2014
Candida fabianii (MBT)	Candida pelliculosa (ID 32C), Candida utilis (ID 32C)	Svobodova et al,[10] 2016
Candida guilliermondii (MBT)	C famata (API 20C AUX, VITEK 2)	Fatania et al,[5] 2015; Chao et al,[9] 2014
Candida intermedia (MBT)	C famata (Microscan)	Ceballos-Garzon et al,[6] 2019
Candida metapsilosis (MBT)	Candida parapsilosis (Microscan)	Ceballos-Garzon et al,[6] 2019
Candida nivariensis (MBT)	Candida glabrata (Microscan, VITEK 2, Phoenix Yeast ID)	Ceballos-Garzon et al,[6] 2019; Chao et al,[9] 2014
Candida orthopsilosis (MBT)	C parapsilosis (VITEK 2, Microscan)	Ceballos-Garzon et al,[6] 2019; Garza-Gonzalez et al,[8] 2020
Candida tropicalis (MBT)	Candida viswanathii (Phoenix Yeast ID)	Chao et al,[9] 2014
Candida zeylanoides (MBT)	Saccharomyces cerevisiae (Phoenix Yeast ID, VITEK 2), Trichosporon asahii (Phoenix Yeast ID, VITEK 2)	Chao et al,[9] 2014
Cryptococcus gattii (MBT)	Cryptococcus neoformans (Microscan)	Ceballos-Garzon et al,[6] 2019
Saprochaete clavata (SARAMIS)	Geotrichum capitatum (VITEK 2)	Lo Cascio et al,[7] 2020

Similarly, MBT and Microscan, an automated biochemical-based testing platform, had a 93.6% concordance when challenged with 498 yeast isolates.[6] Overwhelmingly, most yeast misidentifications that are ultimately corrected by the use of MALDI-TOF MS are attributable to cryptic or recently emerging species, which tend to display higher minimum inhibitory concentrations (MICs) to antifungal agents. One such yeast is *Saprochaete clavata* (formerly *Geotrichum clavatum*), which is intrinsically resistant to echinocandins and fluconazole and was the cause of a cluster of fungemia in hospitalized hematology patients.[7]

Rigorous database representation is a key factor for MALDI-TOF MS success. RUO databases are available for Bruker MBT (RUO) and VITEK MS (SARAMIS) in addition to each manufacturer's FDA-cleared database. In the United States, many laboratories opt to use the FDA-cleared database only because of the significant regulatory requirements to validate an RUO database in a clinical setting. The limitations of relying solely on an approved database, however, was highlighted in 2016 with the rapid emergence of *Candida auris* as a global public health threat. The lack of *C auris* representation in FDA-cleared databases at the time and the misidentification by various phenotypic platforms (see **Table 1**) was concerning because almost all *C auris* isolates were resistant to fluconazole and elevated MICs to voriconazole and amphotericin B had also been reported.[11] Several groups developed their own in-house supplemental databases at the time[12–14] because FDA clearance of updated MBT and VITEK MS databases containing *C auris* became available only mid-to-late 2018, 2 years after identification of what became a global outbreak. An external quality assessment of 47 Dutch laboratories in 2019 showed that only 74% of laboratories could correctly identify *C auris*.[15] This finding is concerning, because most of the misidentifications were attributed to use of older VITEK MS (pre-Knowledgebase 3.2) versions; thus, highlighting the importance for maintaining up-to-date databases and/or reflexing appropriately to additional tests, such as sequencing.

Direct head-to-head comparisons of the MALDI-TOF MS systems for yeast identification generally lean toward better performance of the Bruker MBT compared with VITEK MS[9,16–19]; however, older versions of VITEK MS were studied and analysis focused on cryptic species including *C nivariensis*, *C bracarensis*, *C metapsilosis*, and *C orthopsilosis*. Others, however, have reported comparable performance between Bruker MBT and VITEK MS,[20–23] whereas one group reported better performance of VITEK MS compared with Bruker MBT.[24] The variability across the literature highlights the significant impact of organism challenge sets on performance assessment and emphasizes the need for updated literature that compares current database versions.

RUO databases, such as SARAMIS, have proven useful on multiple occasions where VITEK MS failed to identify *S clavata*,[7] *C glabrata* complex,[25] and *C parapsilosis* complex.[9] However, numerous authors have published better success with MALDI-TOF MS after developing in-house databases to supplement that of the manufacturer including uncommon *Cryptococcus* species, foodborne yeasts, environmental yeasts, and rare *Candida* species.[14,19,26–33] Supplemental databases have also enabled clean differentiation and identification of *Cryptococcus neoformans* and *Cryptococcus gattii* for Bruker MBT and SARAMIS.[32,34]

The requirement for full protein extraction (also known as tube extraction) for yeast identification by MALDI-TOF MS is controversial. Tube extraction, a process by which the organism is lysed and proteins are extracted using a solvent system containing formic acid and acetonitrile, leads to cleaner spectra and better identification scores, and is safer from a biohazard perspective. Full protein extraction was the method initially recommended by Bruker Scientific and BioMerieux on release of MALDI-TOF MS on the clinical market. The method takes only minutes, but the need to improve workflow efficiency and increase throughput in the clinical laboratory led to the use of direct on-plate extraction whereby the organism is smeared onto the target plate followed by matrix (with or without the addition of formic acid). Recently, a large multicenter European study (10 centers, 1511 yeast isolates) that compared different extraction methods showed that Bruker's direct deposition method without formic acid extraction resulted in only 23.16% correct identifications compared with full tube extraction, which yielded significantly better results (78.23%).[35] This finding has been echoed by others in the field for *C auris* and *C neoformans*.[22,36]

Another area of interest for Bruker MBT users has been the lowering of cutoff scores for species- and genus-level identification. Bruker MBT software uses a logarithmic score between 0 and 3 to weight the confidence of a spectral identification. According to manufacturer's cutoffs, scores greater than or equal to 2.0 are confident to species level, scores 1.7 to 1.99 are confident for genus level, whereas spectra that score less than 1.7 cannot be accurately identified. One study showed an 87.2% success rate in species-level identification of 117 mostly *Candida* isolates using the manufacturer's cutoff score of greater than or equal to 2.0,[37] whereas others have demonstrated that a drop in threshold to greater than or equal to 1.7 significantly improved performance without compromising accuracy.[14,27,29,35,38,39] The cutoff score chosen by any laboratory is highly dependent on the quality of the extraction method, expanse of the database, and type of test organisms studied. Regardless of the method used, it is important that any process that deviates from the manufacturer's recommendations is thoroughly validated in the clinical setting before implementing for patient care.

Overall, MALDI-TOF MS has demonstrated successful identification for most yeast isolates. Early reports rightfully highlighted deficiencies in manufacturer's databases for identification of cryptic and emerging yeast species. Although current databases are more expansive with organism representation, variations among strains of the same species may not necessarily guarantee 100% successful identification.[6,24,40] In-house developed databases can improve performance significantly, and are a useful stop gap measure for rapid response to emerging pathogens if rigorously validated and interpreted with care.

MATRIX-ASSISTED LASER DESORPTION IONIZATION TIME-OF-FLIGHT MASS SPECTROMETRY FOR MOLD IDENTIFICATION

Over the last decade, MALDI-TOF MS for accurate mold identification has become the inevitable quest in clinical laboratories given the growing number of recognized fungal pathogens, the emergence of cryptic species with atypical resistance patterns, and the dwindling numbers of laboratorians with skilled mycologic expertise. Although numerous groups have demonstrated successful implementation of MALDI-TOF MS for mold identification into the routine laboratory workflow,[41–43] few laboratories (at least in the United States), have chosen to use this technology for molds because of a series of nonstandardized processes including culture methods, extraction methods, databases, and acquisition methods. The following section summarizes these areas of concern, and guides readers on important considerations when interpreting the literature and when implementing MALDI-TOF MS for routine mold identification in the clinical setting.

Accurate species-level identification of molds has become an important diagnostic tool for patient management because of the emergence of cryptic azole-resistant species, such as *Aspergillus calidoustus* and *Aspergillus lentulus*, which are morphologically similar to *Aspergillus ustus* and *Aspergillus fumigatus*, respectively. When compared with traditional morphologic identification, Gautier and colleagues[44] reported that implementation of MALDI-TOF MS led to a significant improvement in species-level mold identification from 78.2% to 98.1%, and a marked reduction in misidentification rates from 9.8% to 1.2%. Similar findings have been reported by others[45–47] including accurate differentiation within the *Aspergillus niger* clade whereby *Aspergillus tubingensis* exhibited decreased azole susceptibility[48] and accurate identification of *Rasamsonia argillaceae*, which is often misidentified as *Paecilomyces* based on similar morphologic characteristics.[49]

The history of MALDI-TOF MS for mold identification is complex and consists of a culmination of various standardization issues. Early studies focused on the Bruker MBT because it was the first instrument launched into the clinical market with an RUO database. Given the lack of robust mold representation, Cassagne and colleagues[42] were the first in 2011 to design an in-house mold database consisting of 143 strains. In this landmark study, prospective analysis of 197 clinical isolates extracted from solid media resulted in an 87% correct species-level identification, and identification failure was attributed to a lack of organism representation in the database.[42] In that study, each extract was spotted in quadruplicate and the authors applied an algorithm whereby at least three of the four deposits corresponded to the same species with at least one replicate scoring greater than or equal to 1.9. This algorithm has since been widely adopted in other European centers.[44]

In the United States, a different mold MALDI-TOF MS database developed by Lau and colleagues[41] had published in 2013 consisting of 294 strains encompassing 76 genera and 152 species. In this study, blinded analysis of 421 clinical isolates from solid media demonstrated 88.9% species-level identification, while maintaining the manufacturer's cutoff score of greater than or equal to 2.0.[41] Testing was conducted in duplicate spots. Spectral analysis against Bruker's RUO and FilFungal databases at the time had 0.7% and 16.2% sensitivity, respectively, for species-level identification; and 48.4% of isolates failed to identify with the FilFungal database despite having spectral representation.[41] Discussion later highlights that this poor performance against the FilFungal database was likely attributed to spectra acquired from growth on solid media (National Institutes of Health [NIH] method) as opposed to liquid media (Bruker MBT method).

In the years since, a considerable number of publications describing the development of in-house supplemental mold databases have emerged. These have encompassed a variety of molds and have been built on Bruker MBT[50–68] and VITEK MS/SARAMIS systems.[69–73] In every single study, the in-house developed database performed better than the manufacturer's database alone. The most impressive database to be released in recent years has been the freely accessible, World Wide Web–based application Mass Spectrometry Identification (MSI) platform, developed by Normand and colleagues.[50] On its release in 2017, the MSI consisted of 11,851 spectra (938 fungal species and 246 fungal genera) and has been continuously updated since that time. In addition to demonstrating outstanding performance for mold identification from solid media (87.35% MSI vs 39.76% Bruker MBT), the authors were able to provide mass access globally to laboratories that had previously limited access to in-house built databases.[50] Others have also demonstrated excellent performance of the MSI database across clinical and veterinary fields.[47,74–76] At this time, the MSI database is only compatible with spectra acquired from the Bruker MBT platform.

The culture process and extraction method of molds for MALDI-TOF MS have been areas of high variability in the literature. Most studies describing the development and validation of in-house databases, and the VITEK MS method, support the testing of molds grown on solid media because this follows routine clinical mycology processes. However, because of the natural heterogeneity of mold isolates and hence generated spectra, it is recommended that databases hold multiple mass spectral profiles for a single strain to increase the likelihood for identification.[77] The VITEK MS protocol consists of full protein extraction of conidia harvested from growth of molds on solid media. Numerous studies of the VITEK MS for mold identification, including multicenter evaluations, have demonstrated excellent performance ranging between 76.8% and 91%,[43,49,71,78] although improvement in the representation of cryptic *Aspergillus* species is warranted.[71]

In contrast, the Bruker MBT FilFungal database was developed using mold subcultured into liquid broth, which is an uncommon work practice in clinical mycology laboratories. Use of liquid broths was applied to achieve uniform consistency of mycelium, leading to acquisition of more standardized and cleaner spectra, thus overcoming the natural heterogeneity of mold and spectral differences observed when testing isolates directly from solid media.[79] Performance of the FilFungal database following cultivation in liquid media results varies considerably (15.4%–94.5%) for species-level identification across studies.[45,80,81]

Unfortunately, there are no studies that directly compare the performance of the manufacturer's methods and databases alone for mold identification (ie, Bruker MBT liquid cultivation method against FilFungal database, and VITEK MS solid media cultivation against Knowledgebase 3.2). There are, however, two studies that compare both systems and databases from growth on solid media. These modified head-to-head comparisons show an overwhelmingly better performance of the VITEK MS compared with Bruker MBT for mold identification from solid media.[76,82]

Given the variable performance of MALDI-TOF MS for mold identification in the literature, multicenter studies have become the key toward addressing development of a standardized process. Four groups have made headway in this area. The first study by Normand and colleagues[50] showed wide interlaboratory performance for mold identification across five European centers, two different databases (MSI and Bruker MBT), and different cutoff scores. In Canada, Stein and colleagues[47] compared three different databases and also found high interlaboratory variability among three clinical laboratories. These authors reported that the highest and lowest scores were consistently obtained by the same laboratory suggesting instrument variability or inherent reproducibility problems.[47] One could hypothesize that the high interlaboratory variability reported by these two studies may be attributable to variations in test isolates between laboratories for prospective clinical analysis. However, a large multicenter study published by Lau and colleagues[83] in 2019 demonstrated a wide range in performance (33%–77%) across eight different testing centers analyzing 80 identical isolates using the routine Bruker MBT acquisition program against the NIH database. Adjustment of key parameters in the acquisition program, along with optimized instrument maintenance, significantly improved performance for most centers.[83] Following this study, Bruker Scientific announced release of an updated software module (version 3.0) that contained adjusted acquisition parameters specifically to improve mold identification rates. Surprisingly, issues with interlaboratory agreement have only been associated with Bruker MBT platforms; one multicenter study conducted on VITEK MS showed good reproducibility between testing sites.[43] More studies are needed in this area to evaluate the extent of improving interlaboratory agreement based on modified acquisition parameters. However, the findings thus far significantly advance the likelihood for successful implementation of MALDI-TOF MS in laboratories for routine mold identification.

Other variables, such as extraction methods, have also been studied; however, it is abundantly clear that full protein extraction (with or without mechanical disruption) rather than direct plate deposition produces far superior spectra and better-quality identification.[68,82,84] Research into a new media formulation called ID FUNGI plate (Conidia, Quincieux, France) is making recent headlines because it uses a transparent low-adherence membrane across the agar surface that allows for clean mold harvest without interference from the media. Early studies suggest that ID FUNGI plate performs better than conventional media for mold identification on Bruker MBT and against a variety of databases including FilFungal, NIH Database, and MSI Database.[75,85–87] Some also showed successful identification of mold following direct deposition.[86,87] Similar to yeast studies, lowering the cutoff score for Bruker MBT to greater than or equal to 1.7 has been used by several group to improve mold identification without compromising in accuracy.[45,52,58,60,64,66,68,76,80,88]

Overall, significant advances have been made over the last decade to highlight the clinical utility of MALDI-TOF MS for mold identification. It is hoped that key findings regarding acquisition programs and the availability of free online databases, such as

MSI, will make mold identification by MALDI-TOF MS a real and feasible platform across many clinical laboratories.

MATRIX-ASSISTED LASER DESORPTION IONIZATION TIME-OF-FLIGHT MASS SPECTROMETRY FOR FUNGAL IDENTIFICATION DIRECTLY FROM POSITIVE BLOOD CULTURE BOTTLES

Early and accurate detection of fungal bloodstream infections still remains challenging. Rapid identification directly from a positive blood bottle has demonstrated significant improvement in patient outcomes through the timely initiation of appropriate and targeted antimicrobial therapy. Bal and McGill[89] studied 74 patients with candidemia and showed that appropriateness of therapy was significantly higher for the rapid identification (MALDI-TOF MS) group (90.9%) compared with the conventional identification group (62.2%), which also resulted in more than £10,000 cost savings within the first 3 days of treatment. Similarly, de Almeida and coworkers[90] reported that five of seven patients with fungemia had targeted antifungal therapy guided by MALDI-TOF MS species identification directly from positive blood cultures.

Sample preparation and cleanup is critical for ensuring quality spectra and good identification results. To that end, various sample processing methods for red blood cell lysis and removal of inhibitors before MALDI-TOF MS have been evaluated. The Sepsityper kit from Bruker Scientific uses a series of washes for cell lysis and cleanup, resulting in a pellet that can then be chemically extracted following the routine formic acid and acetonitrile process. This method,[89,91] and those applied by others including saponin extraction[92] and sodium dodecyl sulfate lytic extraction,[90] have resulted in only moderate performance for the detection of yeasts directly from positive blood cultures. Short-term incubation of the subculture for 4 to 6 hours did not improve performance even when a lowered threshold of 1.7 was applied,[91,93] although Florio and colleagues[94] reported 100% concordance in identifying yeasts from 17 positive blood cultures, including polymicrobial cultures, while maintaining the manufacturer's threshold of 2.0. In addition to lowering the threshold, multiple spots (eg, quadruplicate), full chemical protein extraction, and RUO databases may need to be applied to improve the performance rate of MALDI-TOF MS for fungal identification directly from positive blood cultures. Regardless of which method is chosen, it is critical that laboratories validate the method to ensure consistent and reliable results. In January 2021, Bruker Scientific announced FDA approval of the Sepsityper kit, which includes detection of bacteria and yeasts. This may assist in interlaboratory standardization and a willingness to implement such tests in the clinical setting to benefit patient care.

MATRIX-ASSISTED LASER DESORPTION IONIZATION TIME-OF-FLIGHT MASS SPECTROMETRY FOR ANTIFUNGAL RESISTANCE DETECTION IN YEASTS AND MOLDS

It is clear that MALDI-TOF MS has had an overwhelmingly positive impact on patient care and epidemiology through the provision of rapid, accurate, and detailed fungal identification. In recent years, MALDI-TOF MS has been used successfully for the detection of antimicrobial resistance markers in bacteria, even sometimes through the use of the same spectral profile already acquired for organism identification.[95,96] The clinical application of MALDI-TOF MS for predicting antifungal susceptibility profiles, however, is still in its infancy, although early research has shown some promise.

The MBT ASTRA method, a supplemental software available by Bruker Scientific and designed originally for resistance detection in bacteria, has been applied by some groups for antifungal resistance detection. The MBT ASTRA method involves the comparison of spectral profiles obtained from an isolate exposed and not exposed to an antimicrobial. Through computational analysis, shifts detected in the spectral profile of the isolate exposed to the antimicrobial may indicate resistance or susceptibility to that agent, depending on the pattern observed. The preincubation exposure time is generally short (~3–6 hours), resulting in a method that may be faster, cheaper, and simpler than traditional Clinical and Laboratory Standards Institute testing and/or sequencing for mutation analysis.

With the emergence of echinocandin resistance in *Candida* species, and reliance of echinocandins for first-line therapy for invasive candidiasis, Vatanshenassan and colleagues[97] used MBT ASTRA to evaluate the performance of MALDI-TOF MS to detect echinocandin resistance in *Candida* species. In their proof of principle study, Vatanshenassan and colleagues[97] demonstrated 100% categorical agreement between MBT ASTRA and CLSI broth microdilution for caspofungin susceptibility profiling of *C albicans* (n = 58). A lower categorical agreement was obtained for *C glabrata* (n = 57) resulting in a sensitivity and specificity of 94% and 80%, respectively, between MBT ASTRA and the CLSI broth microdilution. A follow-up study by this same group evaluated MBT ASTRA for the rapid detection of anidulafungin-resistant *C glabrata* isolates directly from positive blood cultures (n = 100).[98] Here, the MBT ASTRA had a sensitivity and specificity of 80% and 95%, respectively, compared with CLSI broth microdilution, and a positive and negative agreement of 100% and 80%, respectively, when MBT ASTRA was compared with sequencing analysis of hot spots in *FKS1* and *FKS2*.

Similar studies have also been conducted for *C albicans* and fluconazole resistance,[99] *Candida tropicalis* and fluconazole resistance,[100] and *C parapsilosis* complex and echinocandin resistance.[101] All of these groups demonstrated moderate to high success rates for MALDI-TOF MS antifungal susceptibility profiling when compared with a reference method. In contrast, Saracli and colleagues[102] showed that results were too variable when MALDI-TOF MS was applied to triazole resistance detection in various *Candida* species, and Vella and colleagues[103] demonstrated assay variability depending on antifungal exposure time during preincubation. More studies are warranted, but the data thus far suggest that MALDI-TOF MS may be a promising tool for some drug/yeast combinations, but more work is required before such testing becomes mainstream. Conversely, MALDI-TOF MS is unlikely to be a favorable alternative for the susceptibility profiling of molds. A single study showed that voriconazole resistance detection in *Aspergillus fumigatus* was possible but offered no advantages to traditional CLSI testing or *CYP51 A* sequence analysis.[104]

SUMMARY

The clinical mycology field has advanced significantly in technological capabilities over the last decade. Accurate species-level identification of yeasts and molds, particularly within species complexes and cryptic organisms, is highly achievable and practical with MALDI-TOF MS. The wide availability of these platforms in diagnostic settings will likely have a significant impact on patient outcomes by enabling more rapid identification and initiation of appropriate therapy. The simplicity of testing and low-cost consumables makes MALDI-TOF MS an ideal platform in low-resource settings.[105] Although this review focused only on Bruker MBT and VITEK MS platforms, other systems including ASTA MicroIDSys system (ASTA Inc,

Seoul, South Korea) and Xiamen Microtyper (Xiamen, China) have shown excellent performance in preliminary studies.[106,107] The current state of the diagnostic clinical mycology laboratory is exciting, and data suggest that there is a promising era ahead toward standardization and wide implementation of MALDI-TOF MS for fungal identification.

CLINICS CARE POINTS

- With minimal organism biomass, MALDI-TOF MS can provide rapid identification of fungi from culture (including directly from blood culture), which can help guide targeted therapeutic response.
- Identification accuracy is highly dependent on database representation. Use of supplemental databases, including curated online databases, should be considered in the laboratory workflow.
- Implementation of MALDI-TOF MS can provide targeted identification of cryptic species that are generally more resistant to antifungals.

DISCLOSURE

This work was supported by the Intramural Research Program of the National Institutes of Health. The content is solely the authors' responsibility and does not represent the official views of the National Institutes of Health.

REFERENCES

1. Wang H, Wang Y, Yang QW, et al. A national survey on fungal infection diagnostic capacity in the clinical mycology laboratories of tertiary care hospitals in China. J Microbiol Immunol Infect 2020;53(6):845–53.
2. Chindamporn A, Chakrabarti A, Li R, et al. Survey of laboratory practices for diagnosis of fungal infection in seven Asian countries: an Asia Fungal Working Group (AFWG) initiative. Med Mycol 2018;56(4):416–25.
3. Westblade LF, Jennemann R, Branda JA, et al. Multicenter study evaluating the Vitek MS system for identification of medically important yeasts. J Clin Microbiol 2013;51(7):2267–72.
4. Westblade LF, Garner OB, MacDonald K, et al. Assessment of reproducibility of matrix-assisted laser desorption ionization-time of flight mass spectrometry for bacterial and yeast identification. J Clin Microbiol 2015;53(7):2349–52.
5. Fatania N, Fraser M, Savage M, et al. Comparative evaluation of matrix-assisted laser desorption ionisation-time of flight mass spectrometry and conventional phenotypic-based methods for identification of clinically important yeasts in a UK-based medical microbiology laboratory. J Clin Pathol 2015;68(12):1040–2.
6. Ceballos-Garzon A, Cortes G, Morio F, et al. Comparison between MALDI-TOF MS and MicroScan in the identification of emerging and multidrug resistant yeasts in a fourth-level hospital in Bogota, Colombia. BMC Microbiol 2019; 19(1):106.
7. Lo Cascio G, Vincenzi M, Soldani F, et al. Outbreak of *Saprochaete clavata* sepsis in hematology patients: combined use of MALDI-TOF and sequencing strategy to identify and correlate the episodes. Front Microbiol 2020;11:84.
8. Garza-Gonzalez E, Camacho-Ortiz A, Rodriguez-Noriega E, et al. Comparison of matrix-assisted laser desorption ionization time-of-flight mass spectrometry

(MALDI-TOF MS) and the Vitek 2 system for routine identification of clinically relevant bacteria and yeast. Ann Clin Lab Sci 2020;50(1):119–27.

9. Chao QT, Lee TF, Teng SH, et al. Comparison of the accuracy of two conventional phenotypic methods and two MALDI-TOF MS systems with that of DNA sequencing analysis for correctly identifying clinically encountered yeasts. PLoS One 2014;9(10):e109376.

10. Svobodova L, Bednarova D, Ruzicka F, et al. High frequency of *Candida fabianii* among clinical isolates biochemically identified as *Candida pelliculosa* and *Candida utilis*. Mycoses 2016;59(4):241–6.

11. Zhu Y, O'Brien B, Leach L, et al. Laboratory analysis of an outbreak of *Candida auris* in New York from 2016 to 2018: impact and lessons learned. J Clin Microbiol 2020;58(4). e01503-19.

12. Ceballos-Garzon A, Amado D, Velez N, et al. Development and validation of an in-house library of Colombian *Candida auris* strains with MALDI-TOF MS to improve yeast identification. J Fungi (Basel) 2020;6(2):72.

13. Bao JR, Master RN, Azad KN, et al. Rapid, accurate identification of *Candida auris* by using a novel matrix-assisted laser desorption ionization-time of flight mass spectrometry (MALDI-TOF MS) Database (Library). J Clin Microbiol 2018;56(4). e01700-17.

14. Ghosh AK, Paul S, Sood P, et al. Matrix-assisted laser desorption ionization time-of-flight mass spectrometry for the rapid identification of yeasts causing bloodstream infections. Clin Microbiol Infect 2015;21(4):372–8.

15. Buil JB, van der Lee HAL, Curfs-Breuker I, et al. External quality assessment evaluating the ability of Dutch clinical microbiological laboratories to identify *Candida auris*. J Fungi (Basel) 2019;5(4).

16. Hou X, Xiao M, Chen SC, et al. Identification and antifungal susceptibility profiles of *Candida nivariensis* and *Candida bracarensis* in a multi-center Chinese collection of yeasts. Front Microbiol 2017;8:5.

17. Zhao Y, Tsang CC, Xiao M, et al. Yeast identification by sequencing, biochemical kits, MALDI-TOF MS and rep-PCR DNA fingerprinting. Med Mycol 2018;56(7):816–27.

18. Wang H, Fan YY, Kudinha T, et al. A comprehensive evaluation of the Bruker Biotyper MS and Vitek MS matrix-assisted laser desorption ionization-time of flight mass spectrometry systems for identification of yeasts, part of the national China hospital invasive fungal surveillance Net (CHIF-NET) study, 2012 to 2013. J Clin Microbiol 2016;54(5):1376–80.

19. Mancini N, De Carolis E, Infurnari L, et al. Comparative evaluation of the Bruker Biotyper and Vitek MS matrix-assisted laser desorption ionization-time of flight (MALDI-TOF) mass spectrometry systems for identification of yeasts of medical importance. J Clin Microbiol 2013;51(7):2453–7.

20. Kim TH, Kweon OJ, Kim HR, et al. Identification of uncommon *Candida* species using commercial identification systems. J Microbiol Biotechnol 2016;26(12):2206–13.

21. Deak E, Charlton CL, Bobenchik AM, et al. Comparison of the Vitek MS and Bruker Microflex LT MALDI-TOF MS platforms for routine identification of commonly isolated bacteria and yeast in the clinical microbiology laboratory. Diagn Microbiol Infect Dis 2015;81(1):27–33.

22. Lee HS, Shin JH, Choi MJ, et al. Comparison of the Bruker Biotyper and VITEK MS matrix-assisted laser desorption/ionization time-of-flight mass spectrometry systems using a formic acid extraction method to identify common and uncommon yeast isolates. Ann Lab Med 2017;37(3):223–30.

23. Jamal WY, Ahmad S, Khan ZU, et al. Comparative evaluation of two matrix-assisted laser desorption/ionization time-of-flight mass spectrometry (MALDI-TOF MS) systems for the identification of clinically significant yeasts. Int J Infect Dis 2014;26:167–70.

24. Porte L, Garcia P, Braun S, et al. Head-to-head comparison of Microflex LT and Vitek MS systems for routine identification of microorganisms by MALDI-TOF mass spectrometry in Chile. PLoS One 2017;12(5):e0177929.

25. Hou X, Xiao M, Chen SC, et al. Identification of *Candida glabrata* complex species: use of Vitek MS((R)) RUO & Bruker ClinproTools((R)). Future Microbiol 2018;13:645–57.

26. Danesi P, Drigo I, Iatta R, et al. MALDI-TOF MS for the identification of veterinary non-*C. neoformans-C. gattii Cryptococcus* spp. isolates from Italy. Med Mycol 2014;52(6):659–66.

27. Quintilla R, Kolecka A, Casaregola S, et al. MALDI-TOF MS as a tool to identify foodborne yeasts and yeast-like fungi. Int J Food Microbiol 2018;266:109–18.

28. Agustini BC, Silva LP, Bloch C Jr, et al. Evaluation of MALDI-TOF mass spectrometry for identification of environmental yeasts and development of supplementary database. Appl Microbiol Biotechnol 2014;98(12):5645–54.

29. Taverna CG, Mazza M, Bueno NS, et al. Development and validation of an extended database for yeast identification by MALDI-TOF MS in Argentina. Med Mycol 2019;57(2):215–25.

30. Kolecka A, Khayhan K, Groenewald M, et al. Identification of medically relevant species of arthroconidial yeasts by use of matrix-assisted laser desorption ionization-time of flight mass spectrometry. J Clin Microbiol 2013;51(8): 2491–500.

31. Honnavar P, Ghosh AK, Paul S, et al. Identification of *Malassezia* species by MALDI-TOF MS after expansion of database. Diagn Microbiol Infect Dis 2018; 92(2):118–23.

32. Siqueira LPM, Gimenes VMF, de Freitas RS, et al. Evaluation of Vitek MS for differentiation of *Cryptococcus neoformans* and *Cryptococcus gattii* Genotypes. J Clin Microbiol 2019;57(1). e01282-18.

33. de Almeida JN Jr, Favero Gimenes VM, Francisco EC, et al. Evaluating and improving Vitek MS for identification of clinically relevant species of *Trichosporon* and the closely related genera *Cutaneotrichosporon* and *Apiotrichum*. J Clin Microbiol 2017;55(8):2439–44.

34. Posteraro B, Vella A, Cogliati M, et al. Matrix-assisted laser desorption ionization-time of flight mass spectrometry-based method for discrimination between molecular types of *Cryptococcus neoformans* and *Cryptococcus gattii*. J Clin Microbiol 2012;50(7):2472–6.

35. Normand AC, Gabriel F, Riat A, et al. Optimization of MALDI-ToF mass spectrometry for yeast identification: a multicenter study. Med Mycol 2020;58(5): 639–49.

36. Mizusawa M, Miller H, Green R, et al. Can multidrug-resistant *Candida auris* be reliably identified in clinical microbiology laboratories? J Clin Microbiol 2017; 55(2):638–40.

37. Turhan O, Ozhak-Baysan B, Zaragoza O, et al. Evaluation of MALDI-TOF-MS for the identification of yeast isolates causing bloodstream infection. Clin Lab 2017; 63(4):699–703.

38. Cassagne C, Normand AC, Bonzon L, et al. Routine identification and mixed species detection in 6,192 clinical yeast isolates. Med Mycol 2016;54(3): 256–65.

39. Fraser M, Brown Z, Houldsworth M, et al. Rapid identification of 6328 isolates of pathogenic yeasts using MALDI-ToF MS and a simplified, rapid extraction procedure that is compatible with the Bruker Biotyper platform and database. Med Mycol 2016;54(1):80–8.

40. Taverna CG, Cordoba S, Vivot M, et al. Reidentification and antifungal susceptibility profile of *Candida guilliermondii* and *Candida famata* clinical isolates from a culture collection in Argentina. Med Mycol 2019;57(3):314–23.

41. Lau AF, Drake SK, Calhoun LB, et al. Development of a clinically comprehensive database and a simple procedure for identification of molds from solid media by matrix-assisted laser desorption ionization-time of flight mass spectrometry. J Clin Microbiol 2013;51(3):828–34.

42. Cassagne C, Ranque S, Normand AC, et al. Mould routine identification in the clinical laboratory by matrix-assisted laser desorption ionization time-of-flight mass spectrometry. PLoS One 2011;6(12). e28425.

43. Rychert J, Slechta ES, Barker AP, et al. Multicenter evaluation of the Vitek MS v3.0 system for the identification of filamentous fungi. J Clin Microbiol 2018; 56(2). e01353-17.

44. Gautier M, Ranque S, Normand AC, et al. Matrix-assisted laser desorption ionization time-of-flight mass spectrometry: revolutionizing clinical laboratory diagnosis of mould infections. Clin Microbiol Infect 2014;20(12):1366–71.

45. Schulthess B, Ledermann R, Mouttet F, et al. Use of the Bruker MALDI Biotyper for identification of molds in the clinical mycology laboratory. J Clin Microbiol 2014;52(8):2797–803.

46. Ranque S, Normand AC, Cassagne C, et al. MALDI-TOF mass spectrometry identification of filamentous fungi in the clinical laboratory. Mycoses 2014; 57(3):135–40.

47. Stein M, Tran V, Nichol KA, et al. Evaluation of three MALDI-TOF mass spectrometry libraries for the identification of filamentous fungi in three clinical microbiology laboratories in Manitoba, Canada. Mycoses 2018;61(10):743–53.

48. D'Hooge E, Becker P, Stubbe D, et al. Black aspergilli: a remaining challenge in fungal taxonomy? Med Mycol 2019;57(6):773–80.

49. McMullen AR, Wallace MA, Pincus DH, et al. Evaluation of the Vitek MS matrix-assisted laser desorption ionization-time of flight mass spectrometry system for identification of clinically relevant filamentous fungi. J Clin Microbiol 2016;54(8): 2068–73.

50. Normand AC, Becker P, Gabriel F, et al. Validation of a new web application for identification of fungi by use of matrix-assisted laser desorption ionization-time of flight mass spectrometry. J Clin Microbiol 2017;55(9):2661–70.

51. Sleiman S, Halliday CL, Chapman B, et al. Performance of matrix-assisted laser desorption ionization-time of flight mass spectrometry for identification of *Aspergillus*, *Scedosporium*, and *Fusarium* spp. in the Australian clinical setting. J Clin Microbiol 2016;54(8):2182–6.

52. Triest D, Stubbe D, De Cremer K, et al. Use of matrix-assisted laser desorption ionization-time of flight mass spectrometry for identification of molds of the *Fusarium* genus. J Clin Microbiol 2015;53(2):465–76.

53. Chen YS, Liu YH, Teng SH, et al. Evaluation of the matrix-assisted laser desorption/ionization time-of-flight mass spectrometry Bruker Biotyper for identification of *Penicillium marneffei*, *Paecilomyces* species, *Fusarium solani*, *Rhizopus* species, and *Pseudallescheria boydii*. Front Microbiol 2015;6:679.

54. Paul S, Singh P, Sharma S, et al. MALDI-TOF MS-based identification of melanized fungi is faster and reliable after the expansion of in-house database. Proteomics Clin Appl 2019;13(3):e1800070.
55. Hedayati MT, Taghizadeh-Armaki M, Zarrinfar H, et al. Discrimination of *Aspergillus flavus* from *Aspergillus oryzae* by matrix-assisted laser desorption/ionisation time-of-flight (MALDI-TOF) mass spectrometry. Mycoses 2019;62(12):1182–8.
56. Krajaejun T, Lohnoo T, Jittorntam P, et al. Assessment of matrix-assisted laser desorption ionization-time of flight mass spectrometry for identification and biotyping of the pathogenic oomycete *Pythium insidiosum*. Int J Infect Dis 2018;77:61–7.
57. Shao J, Wan Z, Li R, et al. Species identification and delineation of pathogenic mucorales by matrix-assisted laser desorption ionization-time of flight mass spectrometry. J Clin Microbiol 2018;56(4). e01886-17.
58. Becker PT, de Bel A, Martiny D, et al. Identification of filamentous fungi isolates by MALDI-TOF mass spectrometry: clinical evaluation of an extended reference spectra library. Med Mycol 2014;52(8):826–34.
59. Singh A, Singh PK, Kumar A, et al. Molecular and matrix-assisted laser desorption ionization-time of flight mass spectrometry-based characterization of clinically significant melanized fungi in India. J Clin Microbiol 2017;55(4):1090–103.
60. Valero C, Buitrago MJ, Gago S, et al. A matrix-assisted laser desorption/ionization time of flight mass spectrometry reference database for the identification of *Histoplasma capsulatum*. Med Mycol 2018;56(3):307–14.
61. Del Chierico F, Masotti A, Onori M, et al. MALDI-TOF MS proteomic phenotyping of filamentous and other fungi from clinical origin. J Proteomics 2012;75(11):3314–30.
62. Vidal-Acuna MR, Ruiz-Perez de Pipaon M, Torres-Sanchez MJ, et al. Identification of clinical isolates of *Aspergillus*, including cryptic species, by matrix assisted laser desorption ionization time-of-flight mass spectrometry (MALDI-TOF MS). Med Mycol 2018;56(7):838–46.
63. Tartor YH, Abo Hashem ME, Enany S. Towards a rapid identification and a novel proteomic analysis for dermatophytes from human and animal dermatophytosis. Mycoses 2019;62(12):1116–26.
64. Karabicak N, Karatuna O, Ilkit M, et al. Evaluation of the Bruker matrix-assisted laser desorption-ionization time-of-flight mass spectrometry (MALDI-TOF MS) system for the identification of clinically important dermatophyte species. Mycopathologia 2015;180(3–4):165–71.
65. Calderaro A, Motta F, Montecchini S, et al. Identification of dermatophyte species after implementation of the in-house MALDI-TOF MS database. Int J Mol Sci 2014;15(9):16012–24.
66. da Cunha KC, Riat A, Normand AC, et al. Fast identification of dermatophytes by MALDI-TOF/MS using direct transfer of fungal cells on ground steel target plates. Mycoses 2018;61(9):691–7.
67. Theel ES, Hall L, Mandrekar J, et al. Dermatophyte identification using matrix-assisted laser desorption ionization-time of flight mass spectrometry. J Clin Microbiol 2011;49(12):4067–71.
68. Zvezdanova ME, Escribano P, Ruiz A, et al. Increased species-assignment of filamentous fungi using MALDI-TOF MS coupled with a simplified sample processing and an in-house library. Med Mycol 2019;57(1):63–70.
69. Quero L, Courault P, Celliere B, et al. Application of MALDI-TOF MS to species complex differentiation and strain typing of food related fungi: case studies with

Aspergillus section *Flavi* species and *Penicillium roqueforti* isolates. Food Microbiol 2020;86:103311.

70. Quero L, Girard V, Pawtowski A, et al. Development and application of MALDI-TOF MS for identification of food spoilage fungi. Food Microbiol 2019;81:76–88.

71. Americo F, Machado Siqueira L, Del Negro G, et al. Evaluating VITEK MS for the identification of clinically relevant *Aspergillus* species. Med Mycol 2020;58(3):322–7.

72. De Respinis S, Monnin V, Girard V, et al. Matrix-assisted laser desorption ionization-time of flight (MALDI-TOF) mass spectrometry using the Vitek MS system for rapid and accurate identification of dermatophytes on solid cultures. J Clin Microbiol 2014;52(12):4286–92.

73. Nenoff P, Erhard M, Simon JC, et al. MALDI-TOF mass spectrometry: a rapid method for the identification of dermatophyte species. Med Mycol 2013;51(1):17–24.

74. Becker P, Normand AC, Vanantwerpen G, et al. Identification of fungal isolates by MALDI-TOF mass spectrometry in veterinary practice: validation of a web application. J Vet Diagn Invest 2019;31(3):471–4.

75. Heireman L, Patteet S, Steyaert S. Performance of the new ID-fungi plate using two types of reference libraries (Bruker and MSI) to identify fungi with the Bruker MALDI Biotyper. Med Mycol 2020;58(7):946–57.

76. Dupont D, Normand AC, Persat F, et al. Comparison of matrix-assisted laser desorption ionization time of flight mass spectrometry (MALDI-TOF MS) systems for the identification of moulds in the routine microbiology laboratory. Clin Microbiol Infect 2019;25(7):892–7.

77. Normand AC, Cassagne C, Ranque S, et al. Assessment of various parameters to improve MALDI-TOF MS reference spectra libraries constructed for the routine identification of filamentous fungi. BMC Microbiol 2013;13:76.

78. Pinheiro D, Monteiro C, Faria MA, et al. Vitek((R)) MS v3.0 system in the identification of filamentous fungi. Mycopathologia 2019;184(5):645–51.

79. Paul S, Singh P, Rudramurthy SM, et al. Matrix-assisted laser desorption/ionization-time of flight mass spectrometry: protocol standardization and database expansion for rapid identification of clinically important molds. Future Microbiol 2017;12:1457–66.

80. Li Y, Wang H, Hou X, et al. Identification by matrix-assisted laser desorption ionization-time of flight mass spectrometry and antifungal susceptibility testing of non-*Aspergillus* molds. Front Microbiol 2020;11:922.

81. Park JH, Shin JH, Choi MJ, et al. Evaluation of matrix-assisted laser desorption/ionization time-of-fight mass spectrometry for identification of 345 clinical isolates of *Aspergillus* species from 11 Korean hospitals: comparison with molecular identification. Diagn Microbiol Infect Dis 2017;87(1):28–31.

82. Sun Y, Guo J, Chen R, et al. Multicenter evaluation of three different MALDI-TOF MS systems for identification of clinically relevant filamentous fungi. Med Mycol 2020;59(1):81–6.

83. Lau AF, Walchak RC, Miller HB, et al. Multicenter study demonstrates standardization requirements for mold identification by MALDI-TOF MS. Front Microbiol 2019;10:2098.

84. L'Ollivier C, Ranque S. MALDI-TOF-based dermatophyte identification. Mycopathologia 2017;182(1–2):183–92.

85. Cardot Martin E, Renaux C, Catherinot E, et al. Rapid identification of fungi from respiratory samples by Bruker Biotyper matrix-assisted laser desorption/

ionisation time-of-flight using ID-FUNGI plates. Eur J Clin Microbiol Infect Dis 2020;40(2):391–5.

86. Sacheli R, Henri AS, Seidel L, et al. Evaluation of the new ID-FUNGI plates medium from Conidia for MALDI-TOF MS identification of filamentous fungi and comparison with conventional methods as identification tool for dermatophytes from nails, hair and skin samples. Mycoses 2020;63(10):1115–27.

87. Robert MG, Romero C, Dard C, et al. Evaluation of ID FUNGI plates medium for identification of molds by MALDI Biotyper. J Clin Microbiol 2020;58(5).

88. Normand AC, Cassagne C, Gautier M, et al. Decision criteria for MALDI-TOF MS-based identification of filamentous fungi using commercial and in-house reference databases. BMC Microbiol 2017;17(1):25.

89. Bal AM, McGill M. Rapid species identification of *Candida* directly from blood culture broths by Sepsityper-MALDI-TOF mass spectrometry: impact on antifungal therapy. J R Coll Physicians Edinb 2018;48(2):114–9.

90. de Almeida JNJ, Sztajnbok J, da Silva ARJ, et al. Rapid identification of moulds and arthroconidial yeasts from positive blood cultures by MALDI-TOF mass spectrometry. Med Mycol 2016;54(8):885–9.

91. Fang C, Zhou Z, Li J, et al. Rapid identification of microorganisms from positive blood cultures in pediatric patients by MALDI-TOF MS: Sepsityper kit versus short-term subculture. J Microbiol Methods 2020;172:105894.

92. Hu YL, Hsueh SC, Ding GS, et al. Applicability of an in-house saponin-based extraction method in Bruker Biotyper matrix-assisted laser desorption/ionization time-of-flight mass spectrometry system for identifying bacterial and fungal species in positively flagged pediatric VersaTREK blood cultures. J Microbiol Immunol Infect 2020;53(6):916–24.

93. Bellanger AP, Gbaguidi-Haore H, Liapis E, et al. Rapid identification of *Candida* sp. by MALDI-TOF mass spectrometry subsequent to short-term incubation on a solid medium. APMIS 2019;127(4):217–21.

94. Florio W, Cappellini S, Giordano C, et al. A new culture-based method for rapid identification of microorganisms in polymicrobial blood cultures by MALDI-TOF MS. BMC Microbiol 2019;19(1):267.

95. Lau AF, Wang H, Weingarten RA, et al. A rapid matrix-assisted laser desorption ionization-time of flight mass spectrometry-based method for single-plasmid tracking in an outbreak of carbapenem-resistant enterobacteriaceae. J Clin Microbiol 2014;52(8):2804–12.

96. Youn JH, Drake SK, Weingarten RA, et al. Clinical performance of a matrix-assisted laser desorption ionization time-of-flight mass spectrometry method for the detection of certain blaKPC-containing plasmids. J Clin Microbiol 2015;54(1):35–42.

97. Vatanshenassan M, Boekhout T, Lass-Florl C, et al. Proof of concept for MBT AS-TRA, a rapid matrix-assisted laser desorption ionization-time of flight mass spectrometry (MALDI-TOF MS)-based method to detect caspofungin resistance in *Candida albicans* and *Candida glabrata*. J Clin Microbiol 2018;56(9). e00420-18.

98. Vatanshenassan M, Arastehfar A, Boekhout T, et al. Anidulafungin susceptibility testing of *Candida glabrata* isolates from blood cultures by the MALDI Biotyper antibiotic (antifungal) susceptibility test rapid assay. Antimicrob Agents Chemother 2019;63(9). e00554-19.

99. Delavy M, Cerutti L, Croxatto A, et al. Machine learning approach for candida albicans fluconazole resistance detection using matrix-assisted laser desorption/ionization time-of-flight mass spectrometry. Front Microbiol 2019;10:3000.

100. Paul S, Singh P, Shamanth AS, et al. Rapid detection of fluconazole resistance in *Candida tropicalis* by MALDI-TOF MS. Med Mycol 2018;56(2):234–41.

101. Roberto AEM, Xavier DE, Vidal EE, et al. Rapid detection of echinocandins resistance by MALDI-TOF MS in *Candida parapsilosis* complex. Microorganisms 2020;8(1).

102. Saracli MA, Fothergill AW, Sutton DA, et al. Detection of triazole resistance among *Candida* species by matrix-assisted laser desorption/ionization-time of flight mass spectrometry (MALDI-TOF MS). Med Mycol 2015;53(7):736–42.

103. Vella A, De Carolis E, Mello E, et al. Potential use of MALDI-ToF mass spectrometry for rapid detection of antifungal resistance in the human pathogen *Candida glabrata*. Sci Rep 2017;7(1):9099.

104. Gitman MR, McTaggart L, Spinato J, et al. Antifungal susceptibility testing of aspergillus spp. by using a composite correlation index (CCI)-based matrix-assisted laser desorption ionization-time of flight mass spectrometry method appears to not offer benefit over traditional broth microdilution testing. J Clin Microbiol 2017; 55(7):2030–4.

105. Sow D, Fall B, Ndiaye M, et al. Usefulness of MALDI-TOF mass spectrometry for routine identification of *Candida* species in a resource-poor setting. Mycopathologia. 2015;180(3–4):173–9.

106. Lee H, Park JH, Oh J, et al. Evaluation of a new matrix-assisted laser desorption/ionization time-of-flight mass spectrometry system for the identification of yeast isolation. J Clin Lab Anal 2019;33(2):e22685.

107. Huang Y, Zhang M, Zhu M, et al. Comparison of two matrix-assisted laser desorption ionization-time of flight mass spectrometry systems for the identification of clinical filamentous fungi. World J Microbiol Biotechnol 2017;33(7):142.

Mass Spectrometry and Microbial Diagnostics in the Clinical Laboratory

Christopher R. Cox, PhD[a],*, Rebecca M. Harris, MD[b]

KEYWORDS

- Microbial mass spectrometry • Microbial profiling • Clinical diagnostics

KEY POINTS

- Mass spectrometry has revolutionized the practice of clinical diagnostic microbiology.
- Microbial protein profiling by matrix-assisted laser desorption/ionization time-of-flight mass spectrometry has achieved widespread adoption because it allows rapid identification of bacteria, mycobacteria, yeast, and molds in less time and at less cost than conventional methods.
- Rapid accurate diagnostics allow physicians to initiate antimicrobial therapies with greater likelihood of success earlier in the treatment course, thereby improving patient outcomes and decreasing costs associated with patient care.
- New innovations in mass spectrometry continue to expand clinical diagnostic capabilities.

INTRODUCTION/HISTORY/DEFINITIONS/BACKGROUND

Introduction

Over the past 10 years, mass spectrometry (MS) has revolutionized the practice of clinical microbiology. Microbial protein profiling via matrix-assisted laser desorption/ionization (MALDI)–time-of-flight (TOF) MS has achieved widespread adoption by laboratories because it allows rapid identification of bacteria, mycobacteria, yeast, and molds in less time and at less cost than conventional methods. The availability of Food and Drug Administration (FDA)-cleared MALDI-TOF systems coupled with the ease of sample preparation inherent to MALDI-TOF analysis has accelerated acceptance of this technology within the clinical laboratory. Rapid and accurate microorganism identification allows physicians to initiate antimicrobial therapies with greater likelihood of success earlier in the treatment course, thereby improving patient outcomes and decreasing costs associated with patient care. Although researchers continue to explore additional applications of MALDI-TOF as well as expand

[a] Cobio Diagnostics, Golden, CO, USA; [b] Infectious Disease Diagnostics Laboratory, Children's Hospital of Philadelphia, 3401 Civic Center Boulevard, Philadelphia, PA 19104, USA
* Corresponding author. 1936 Goldenvue Drive, CO 80401.
E-mail address: crcoxcc@gmail.com

Clin Lab Med 41 (2021) 285–295
https://doi.org/10.1016/j.cll.2021.03.007
0272-2712/21/© 2021 Elsevier Inc. All rights reserved.

capabilities with new innovations in MS and assess their benefit to patient care, these technologies already have established themselves as the standard of care for microbial diagnostics.

BACKGROUND

Conventionally, microorganism identification in the laboratory has relied on biochemical testing, which requires organism isolation and then incubation for days to weeks. Using MS, analysis can be performed directly on monoculture isolates grown on agar growth media or extract of harvested cells. Whole cells or protein extracts produced by suspension of pure microbial colonies in ethanol, formic acid, and acetonitrile are placed on a stainless-steel target plate, which then is overlaid with a matrix, and placed in the MALDI-TOF MS instrument. Within the instrument, the plate is charged to high voltage and a laser is fired at the organism/matrix mixture, which absorbs the energy, resulting in largely intact and ionized biomolecules (primarily highly conserved ribosomal proteins) that are accelerated by an electric field through a TOF tube to a detector, with ions separated based on their mass-to-charge ratio. Resulting mass spectra are compared with a protein profile reference database, and a report of the most likely identity is generated.

DISCUSSION

MS microbial diagnostic identification is performed predominately using MALDI-TOF. There currently are 2 FDA-cleared MALDI-TOF MS identification systems that are used widely: the Bruker Biotyper (Bruker, Billerica, MA) and the bioMérieux VITEK MS (bioMérieux, Marcy-l'Étoile, France). Since FDA clearance in 2013, the manufacturers of both systems have obtained approval for expanded diagnostic capabilities and updated reference databases. Bruker recently has commercialized an add-on called the MBT Sepsityper, based on work by La Scola and Raoult[1] that allows for identification of organisms isolated from blood bottle analysis systems. The Sepsityper is a kit that is utilized with positive blood gas bottles derived from the BD BACTEC (Becton Dickinson, Franklin Lakes, NJ) system. Sepsityper reagents serve to lyse blood cells and enrich putatively detected organisms for subsequent Biotyper identification. Further development led to the recent introduction of the Bruker MBT STAR-Carba and MBT STAR-Cepha IVD kits, which are designed to test for phenotypic antibiotic resistance for specific organisms and antimicrobials. The comparative ease of implementing an FDA-cleared testing system has opened the use of MALDI-TOF with such expansion kits to allow blood-based identification and antimicrobial resistance screening to facilities that cannot feasibly perform the extensive validation needed for a complex laboratory-developed identification system. This also has the added benefit that regularly updated and expanded organism profile databases likewise continue to expand the number of species that can be identified routinely for many laboratories.

Several studies have shown that bacterial and yeast identification by MALDI-TOF is superior to the identification method being replaced[2,3] and generally is associated with reduced turnaround time and overall cost due to lower reagent and labor costs.[4–6]

As outcome-based studies on MALDI-TOF are published, there is increasing evidence that its impact can extend to improving patient care and reducing costs. Available publications have focused on analysis of patients with positive blood cultures, because rapid initiation of appropriate antibiotic therapy in patients with sepsis is known to have a dramatic impact on patient survival.[7]

Early work by Perez and colleagues[8] examined the effect of implementing MALDI-TOF in conjunction with an antimicrobial stewardship program (ASP) on patient care outcomes and health care expenditures for patients with gram-negative bloodstream infections. With an active ASP, therapy can be tailored to the identified species, incorporating antibiogram data on the prevalence of antibiotic resistance within the hospital, instead of utilizing broad-spectrum antibiotic coverage based on a gram stain result, earlier in a patient's treatment course. The patient population examined by Perez and colleagues is an ideal subset likely to experience an impact from such intervention, because mortality due to gram-negative bloodstream infections is high, and empirical antibiotic therapy is more likely to be ineffective. Patients in the study postintervention, compared with preintervention, had significantly shortened hospital stays (eg, 9.3 d vs 11.9 d, respectively) and markedly reduced average hospital costs (eg, $26,162 vs $45,709, respectively). Additional work by Perez and colleagues[9] examined patients with antibiotic-resistant gram-negative bloodstream infections for the same intervention and showed significant improvements in clinical outcome measures, including time to optimal therapy, length of hospital and intensive care unit stays, and all-cause 30-day mortality.

Studies examining additional populations of patients with positive blood cultures continue to add evidence that MALDI-TOF can have a positive impact on patient care and hospital finances. In an analysis of a MALDI-TOF with ASP intervention for patients with blood cultures of gram-positive and gram-negative bacteria and Candida species, Huang and colleagues[10] demonstrated significantly decreased time to optimal therapy, from 90.3 hours to 47.3 hours. A similar study done on a pediatric population found a reduction in time to optimal therapy, from 77 hours to 54.2 hours.[11]

Another study of patients with blood cultures positive for coagulase-negative Staphylococcus, a frequent contaminant, highlighted that benefits may come not only from initiation of appropriate antibiotic therapy but also from decreased duration of unnecessary antibiotics.[12]

A comprehensive cost analysis study by Patel and colleagues[13] examined the impact of MALDI-TOF for rapid organism identification coupled with an active ASP for patients with bloodstream infections due to any microorganism. Despite the initial cost of the instrumentation and additional pharmacy personnel time for stewardship intervention, total hospital costs decreased by an average of $2439 per bloodstream infection, amounting to an estimated annual savings of $2.34 million for the hospital. A significant decrease in 30-day mortality from 21% to 12% also was observed. Active antimicrobial stewardship is essential; the clinical team must act on the diagnostic data for the patient to benefit. This need was explored in a recent publication by Beganovic and colleagues,[14] examining MALDI-TOF alone versus MALDI-TOF combined with ASP. MALDI-TOF plus ASP intervention significantly reduced the time to optimal therapy (43.1 h) compared with use of MALI-TOF alone (75.2 h). These data underscore the importance of interdepartmental collaboration within the hospital to achieve the full benefit of laboratory advancements.

Although the benefits of bacterial and yeast isolate identification by MALDI-TOF are the most clearly established, MALDI-TOF has an actively evolving, expanding role in the clinical laboratory. In addition to bacteria and yeasts, MALDI-TOF can be used to identify both filamentous fungi and mycobacterial isolates. The impact of MALDI-TOF on the routine practice of mycology and mycobacteriology is an active area of investigation.[15–17] With the recent availability of FDA-cleared databases, that impact likely will grow. MALDI-TOF has an additional promising capacity in identification directly from positive blood cultures without subculture.[18,19] This can be performed using a laboratory developed process or commercial purification kits, and the modified workflow further expedites identification of organisms from positive blood cultures.

New and Emerging Mass Spectrometric Approaches With Potential for Microbial Diagnostics

Promising new MS ionization approaches beyond MALDI hold new potential for clinical microbial diagnostics (summarized in **Table 1**). These include metal oxide laser ionization (MOLI), a variation of MALDI, as well as ambient ionization approaches, such as direct analysis in real time (DART) and rapid evaporative ionization MS (REIMS). Liquid-phase ionization techniques, such as electrospray ionization (ESI) and desorption ESI (DESI) also have been applied successfully to microbial analysis.

Metal Oxide Laser Ionization Mass Spectrometry

Microbial protein profiling by MALDI-TOF MS is an increasingly utilized tool for diagnostic bacterial identification. It has quickly gained widespread global adoption in clinical and diagnostic research laboratories for rapid pathogen identification with the Bruker Biotyper and bioMérieux VITEK MS.[20,21] MALDI has improved clinical outcomes through high-throughput pathogen isolate identification while also holding the potential to improve antibiotic stewardship with evolving methods for differentiation of resistant isolates. These current systems, however, although rapid and user friendly, do have some limitations. Notably, protein profile-based MALDI has been found to be problematic for differentiation of closely related clinically significant members of the *Enterobacteriaceae* (eg, *Salmonella* and *Shigella*), the *Acinetobacter calcoaceticus* complex (including *Acinetobacter baumannii*), and *Listeria*.[22] This is thought to occur because some closely related species express many similar if not identical proteins, which are represented in reference spectra in manufacturer databases and among clinical isolates. This can result in the reporting of incorrect identifications or diagnostic failures. To address this drawback, through the development of MOLI MS, other potentially taxonomic microbial biomolecules have been evaluated for diagnostic identification. Another limitation to conventional MALDI, when considering alternative diagnostic targets other than proteins, is that of matrix interference when analyzing small biomolecules, such as fatty acids (at or below 400 m/z). The MALDI matrices typically used for co-ionization of protein analytes occupy the same relative mass range of fatty acids, making conventional MALDI measurement intractable. As such, MOLI lipid analysis allowed for matrix-free analysis of fatty acids MALDI instrumentation without interference.[23]

The MOLI approach exploits the catalytic surface properties of, for instance, the rare earth lanthanides, such as cerium oxide, to perform in situ cleavage of intact microbial lipids into their constituent fatty acids in combination with the energy provided by the MALDI laser. In this way, intact microbial colonies or extracts of colonies are overlain directly on a thin cerium oxide layer applied to a conventional MALDI target plate in place of a traditional aromatic chemical matrix. Lipids are cleaved in situ when exposed to laser irradiation and the resulting fatty acids are ionized and analyzed with a conventional MALDI spectrometer. Cox and colleagues[22,24] investigated MOLI MS lipid-based profiling specifically for identification and differentiation of *Enterobacteriaceae*, *Acinetobacter*, and *Listeria* isolates, which have proved difficult to analyze by protein profiling, suggesting a MOLI lipid-based analysis, either to supplement protein analysis or on its own, may prove superior to the current paradigm of a solely focusing on microbial protein composition. The MIDI Sherlock Gas Chromatography Mass spectrometry (GC MS) system (Midi, Inc., Newark, DE) for analysis of microbial fatty acid methyl esters, although more complex to perform and not widely clinically adopted, has proved for decades that lipid-based diagnostic identification is a viable alternative to genotypic and proteomic approaches.[25]

Table 1
Mass spectrometry platforms currently used for clinical microbial diagnostics

Type	Instrument	Clinical Adoption	Advantages	Disadvantages
MALDI-TOF MS Protein profiling	Bruker Biotyper. bioMérieux VITEK MS	Yes	Phenotypic, accurate, high throughput	Requires minimum overnight pure culture; identification only; no AST; problematic for some closely related phenotypes and filamentous fungi
MALDI-TOF MS Protein profiling	Bruker Sepsityper	Yes	Adapts Biotyper to blood analysis postculture	Requires minimum overnight pure culture
MALDI-TOF MS Protein profiling	Bruker MBT STAR-Carba and MBT STAR-Cepha IVD kits	No	Enables AST coupled with MS	Requires minimum overnight pure culture
MOLI MS lipid/fatty acid profiling	Works with any negative ion capable MALDI	No	Phenotypic, accurate, adaptable, high throughput; capable of providing species and strain-level identification and AST for bacteria and fungi	Requires minimum overnight pure culture
DART	JEOL AccuTOF	No	Minimal sample preparation	Requires minimum overnight pure culture; no AST
REIMS	Waters laser ablation-REIMS iKnife and QToF systems	No	Direct-from-colony analysis; minimal sample preparation; high throughput; strain-level capable	Requires minimum overnight pure culture; no AST
ESI	Abbott IRIDICA BAC BSI (PCR-ESI MS/MS)	No	Minimal sample preparation	Requires minimum overnight pure culture; susceptible to variations in growth media formulation and culture conditions; no AST; requires nuclease-free conditions throughout
DESI	Thermo LCQ ion trap; triple quadrapole GC MS	No	Minimal sample preparation	Requires minimum overnight pure culture; susceptible to variations in growth media formulation and culture conditions; no AST

Metal Oxide Laser Ionization Imaging

MOLI MS most recently has seen application in MS tissue imaging (MOLI MSI). Basu and colleagues[26] demonstrated simultaneous MOLI MSI co-imaging of brain tissue and bacteria. MOLI MSI of normal murine brain tissues in comparison to glioblastoma xenografts showed differentiable fatty acyl species in myelinated and nonmyelinated tissues. The work further showed that MOLI allowed for pathogen detection in these tissues when exposed to *Escherichia coli* pseudoinfection. MOLI imaging revealed localization of bacterial-enriched acyl groups readily differentiated from brain tissue–derived spectra, allowing *in situ* differentiation of bacteria from healthy and cancerous mammalian tissues based on the fatty acid profiles of each.

Direct Analysis in Real Time

The Japan Electron Optics Laboratory (JEOL, Peabody, MA) company has developed a noncontact surface sampling technique for MS or ion mobility spectrometry at atmospheric pressures, termed DART. Conventional ion sources used in MS require the introduction of samples into a high vacuum system. The DART ion source is operated on the front end of the JEOL AccuTOF atmospheric pressure ionization MS to allow for soft ionization resulting in high-resolution MS of gases, liquids, and solids at ambient open-air pressure.[27]

This approach, in addition to being demonstrated for real time analysis of various chemical, explosive, and drug compounds, has been used to profile microbial fatty acids.[28–30] Pierce and colleagues[28] demonstrated the technique with fatty acid methyl esters derived from whole-cell suspensions of *Streptococcus pyogenes*, *E coli*, and *Coxiella burnetii*. Cody and colleagues[29] further advanced the concept with successful DART differentiation of clinical isolates and reference strains, including gram-positive *Bacillus anthracis*, *Clostridium putrefaciens*, vancomycin-resistant *Enterococcus faecalis*, *Listeria monocytogenes*, and *Staphylococcus aureus*, and gram-negative *A baumannii*, *E coli*, *Francisella tularensis*, *Salmonella typhimurium*, and *Yersinia pestis*. Because of its capacity to directly analyze bacteria and fungi, either as colony extracts or in body fluids, DART has the potential for direct-from-specimen analysis of infection, although this has yet to be widely implemented at the clinical level.

Rapid Evaporative Ionization Mass Spectrometry

REIMS is another emerging mass approach with potential for rapid clinical microbial identification. The approach was first developed for real time, in situ interoperative surgical analysis (Waters Corp, Milford, MA) of tissue margins during solid tumor resections with the Waters iKnife for laser ample ablation coupled with the Waters QTof for MS/MS mass analysis.[31] REIMS spectra derived by this method are composed mainly of complex lipids from cellular membranes, which allow histologic specificity that allows differentiation between healthy and cancerous tissues.

REIMS analysis has been adapted similarly, to be performed directly on pure microbial colonies growing on nutrient agar. In this way, isolated single colony morphologies are heated rapidly with a handheld or robotically controlled forceps that houses the REIMS apparatus to thermally lyse cells and produce an aerosol of gas-phase phospholipid ions. Microbial mass spectra are produced by introducing the aerosols into a MS. Resulting spectra are compared with a spectral database for classification. This approach has been used to successfully identify a wide range of clinical bacterial and fungal isolates to the species level, including *S aureus*, *Streptococcus agalactiae* and *Streptococcus pyogenes*, *Citrobacter koseri*, *E coli*, *Klebsiella pneumoniae*, *Proteus mirabilis*, *Pseudomonas aeruginosa*, and *Serratia marcescens*.[32–34]

Electrospray Ionization Mass Spectrometry

ESI is a technique used to ionize a sample by solvating it in a liquid and applying high voltage as it is passed through a nozzle to create an aerosol, which subsequently is analyzed by MS, often with tandem mass analysis. ESI is a soft ionization technique, particularly well-suited for analysis of biological macromolecules that are prone to fragmentation using hard ionization methods. This approach is suitable for interrogation of a wide range of sample types including microbial cultures, clinical swabs (eg, nasal, nasopharyngeal, throat, and skin), or directly from sputum or blood samples, as some examples. The technique also can be applied to analyze environmental samples, such as surface swabs or water samples, food samples, and forensic samples (eg, bone, hair, and teeth).[35,36]

Abbott Molecular Diagnostics (Chicago, IL) commercialized ESI for clinical microbial identification with the Ibis Plex-ID and the IRIDICA BAC BSI assay, which combines polymerase chain reaction (PCR) amplification of species-specific genotypic markers from a wide range of more than 200 bacterial, fungal, and viral isolates.[37–39] Nucleic acids are extracted first, either directly from clinical specimens or from cultivated microbial isolates. The system then performs automated PCR sample preparation and ionization via electrospray. PCR amplicons are analyzed with a TOF mass analyzer, and their base compositions are determined from the resulting mass spectra. Spectra are compared with a database to determine microbial identification. Lack of purity during preparation of samples is a known limitation to this technique and can have a negative impact on outcomes. Thus, as with any molecular amplification–based approach, careful sample preparation is essential and ultraclean DNase or RNase-free sample reagents are required to minimize sample degradation and eliminate background nucleic acid contamination.

Strålin and colleagues[37] recently evaluated the Abbott platform for analysis of positive blood cultures in a multicenter study of 16 US and European hospitals. When analyzing whole-blood samples spiked with known isolates or negative controls, PCR/ESI MS achieved 99.1% true-positive and 97.2% true-negative outcomes. Compared with standard blood culturing practices, PCR/ESI MS produced greater than 94% species specificity against infection-positive patient specimens, which included a range of gram-positive and gram-negatives and *Candida* species. Although currently not clinically adopted, these results suggest future utility for ESI MS combined with molecular diagnosis of bloodstream infections.

Desorption Electrospray Ionization Mass Spectrometry

Similar to ESI MS, DESI MS has also been investigated for bacterial identification. DESI differs from ESI in that the charged electrospray solvent stream is directed at a sample affixed to a charged surface.[40] Rather than solvate the analyte prior to electrospray, during DESI the electrospray solvent is aimed at a surface-absorbed sample at an offset angle relative to the analyte to affect ionization and propel secondary ions off the surface toward a mass analyzer. The analyte surface is charged by applying a voltage to the sample and the analyte is extracted by the solvent, which aerosolizes as charged droplets that evaporate to form ions. Analysis is performed with a DESI-source interfaced to a quadrupole ion trap MS system, such as the Thermo LCQ (Thermo Finnigan, LLC., San Jose, CA).

Meetani and colleagues[41] demonstrated DESI MS with a triple quadrupole ion trap MS for lipid profiling of a range of gram-negative and gram-positive bacteria. This approach was applied to microbial identification because of its capacity as an ambient atmospheric pressure ionization technique, which allows for analysis, much in the same way as MALDI, of intact biomolecules in the low mass range (below 500 Da). A range of gram-positive and gram-negative bacteria were tested, including *Bordetella bronchiseptica*, *Bacillus thuringiensis*, *Bacillus subtilis*, *Enterococcus*, *S aureus*, *E coli*, and *Salmonella typhimurium*, and differentiated based on their individual DESI mass spectral profiles in a low mass range of 50 Da to 500 Da. Positive ion profiles were compared using principal components analysis to investigate reproducibility. Results were shown to be consistent from day to day for analyses conducted over multiday experiments. It was observed, however, that reproducibility was highly dependent on growth media lots and cultivation conditions that would detract from its application in the clinical laboratory. That said, with careful adherence to standard operating procedures for media preparation and microbial growth, direct isolate DESI analysis has the potential for highly accurate microbial identification with minimal sample preparation requirements relative to other MS approaches.

SUMMARY

MS, primarily through MALDI-TOF, is firmly established in the clinical microbiology laboratory. Its utility is clear, and a growing body of research shows the potential for MALDI-TOF implementation to improve treatment outcomes and ultimately benefit patient care. As MALDI-TOF continues to be adopted more widely by hospitals and actively investigated, an increasingly expansive role for its use likely will be seen. With additional applications of MALDI-TOF, and potentially other MS-based systems on the horizon, the future of MS in clinical microbiology is bright and highly collimated. The capacity of new MS approaches, such as MOLI MS, DART, REIMS, and electrospray applications, to allow side-by-side protein, lipid, and other macromolecular analyses with MSs, coupled with its potential for strain-level identification of even the most problematic species, stands to advance MS microbial diagnostics even further in the future.

CLINICS CARE POINTS

- Pathogen identification in the laboratory historically has relied on biochemical testing, which requires organism isolation and then incubation for days to weeks.
- Rapid and accurate microorganism identification allows physicians to initiate antimicrobial therapies with greater likelihood of success earlier in the treatment course, thereby improving patient outcomes and decreasing costs associated with patient care.

DISCLOSURE

The authors have nothing to disclose.

REFERENCES

1. La Scola B, Raoult D. Direct identification of bacteria in positive blood culture bottles by matrix-assisted laser desorption ionisation time-of-flight mass spectrometry. PLoS One 2009;4(11):e8041.
2. Seng P, Drancourt M, Gouriet F, et al. Ongoing revolution in bacteriology: routine identification of bacteria by matrix-assisted laser desorption ionization time-of-flight mass spectrometry. Clin Infect Dis 2009;49(4):543.
3. van Veen SQ, Claas EC, Kuijper EJ. High-throughput identification of bacteria and yeast by matrix-assisted laser desorption ionization-time of flight mass spectrometry in conventional medical microbiology laboratories. J Clin Microbiol 2010;48(3):900.

4. Theparee T, Das S, Thomson RB Jr. Total laboratory automation and matrix-assisted laser desorption ionization-time of flight mass spectrometry improve turnaround times in the clinical microbiology laboratory: a retrospective analysis. J Clin Microbiol 2018;56. e01242-17.
5. Tan KE, Ellis BC, Lee R, et al. Prospective evaluation of a matrix-assisted laser desorption ionization-time of flight mass spectrometry system in a hospital clinical microbiology laboratory for identification of bacteria and yeasts: a bench-by-bench study for assessing the impact on time to identification and cost-effectiveness. J Clin Microbiol 2012;50(10):3301.
6. Seng P, Abat C, Rolain JM, et al. Identification of rare pathogenic bacteria in a clinical microbiology laboratory: impact of matrix-assisted laser desorption ionization-time of flight mass spectrometry. J Clin Microbiol 2013;51(7):2182.
7. Kumar A, Roberts D, Wood KE, et al. Duration of hypotension before initiation of effective antimicrobial therapy is the critical determinant of survival in human septic shock. Crit Care Med 2006;34(6):1589.
8. Perez KK, Olsen RJ, Musick WL, et al. Integrating rapid pathogen identification and antimicrobial stewardship significantly decreases hospital costs. Arch Pathol Lab Med 2013;137(9):1247.
9. Perez KK, Olsen RJ, Musick WL, et al. Integrating rapid diagnostics and antimicrobial stewardship improves outcomes in patients with antibiotic-resistant Gram-negative bacteremia. J Infect 2014;69(3):216.
10. Huang AM, Newton D, Kunapuli A, et al. Impact of rapid organism identification via matrix-assisted laser desorption/ionization time-of-flight combined with antimicrobial stewardship team intervention in adult patients with bacteremia and candidemia. Clin Infect Dis 2013;57(9):1237.
11. Malcolmson C, Ng K, Hughes S, et al. Impact of matrix-assisted laser desorption and ionization time-of-flight and antimicrobial stewardship intervention on treatment of bloodstream infections in hospitalized children. J Pediatr Infect Dis Soc 2017;6(2):178.
12. Nagel JL, Huang AM, Kunapuli A, et al. Impact of antimicrobial stewardship intervention on coagulase-negative *Staphylococcus* blood cultures in conjunction with rapid diagnostic testing. J Clin Microbiol 2014;52(8):2849.
13. Patel TS, Kaakeh R, Nagel JL, et al. Cost analysis of implementing matrix-assisted laser desorption ionization-time of flight mass spectrometry plus real-time antimicrobial stewardship intervention for bloodstream infections. J Clin Microbiol 2017;55(1):60.
14. Beganovic M, Costello M, Wieczorkiewicz SM. Effect of matrix-assisted laser desorption ionization-time of flight mass spectrometry (MALDI-TOF MS) Alone versus MALDI-TOF MS combined with real-time antimicrobial stewardship interventions on time to optimal antimicrobial therapy in patients with positive blood cultures. J Clin Microbiol 2017;55(5):1437.
15. Rodriguez-Sanchez B, Ruiz-Serrano MJ, Ruiz A, et al. Evaluation of MALDI biotyper mycobacteria library v3.0 for Identification of Nontuberculous Mycobacteria. J Clin Microbiol 2016;54(4):1144.
16. Rodriguez-Temporal D, Perez-Risco D, Struzka EA, et al. Impact of updating the MALDI-TOF MS database on the identification of nontuberculous mycobacteria. J Mass Spectrom 2017;52(9):597.
17. Rychert J, Sue Slechta E, Barker AP, et al. Multicenter evaluation of the Vitek MS v3.0 system for the identification of filamentous fungi. J Clin Microbiol 2018;56. e01353-17.

18. Faron ML, Buchan BW, Ledeboer NA. Matrix-assisted desorption ionization time of flight mass spectrometry for the use with positive blood cultures: methodology, performance, and optimization. J Clin Microbiol 2017;55:3328.

19. Osthoff M, Gürtler N, Bassetti S, et al. Impact of MALDI-TOF-MS-based identification directly from positive blood cultures on patient management: a controlled clinical trial. Clin Microbiol Infect 2017;23(2):78.

20. Jamal W, Albert MJ, Rotimi VO. Real-time comparative evaluation of bioMerieux VITEK MS versus Bruker Microflex MS, two matrix-assisted laser desorption-ionization time-of-flight mass spectrometry systems, for identification of clinically significant bacteria. BMC Microbiol 2014;14:289.

21. Kostrzewa M. Application of the MALDI Biotyper to clinical microbiology: progress and potential. Expert Rev Proteomics 2018;15(3):193.

22. Cox CR, Saicheck NR, Jensen KR, et al. Strain level bacterial identification by CeO_2-catalyzed MALDI-TOF MS analysis and comparison to protein-based methods. Nat Scientific Rep 2015;5:10470.

23. McAlpin CR, Voorhees KJ, Corpuz AR, et al. Analysis of lipids: metal oxide laser ionization mass spectrometry. Anal Chem 2012;84(18):7677.

24. Saichek NR, Cox CR, Kim S, et al. Strain-level *Staphylococcus* differentiation by CeO_2-metal oxide laser ionization mass spectrometry fatty acid profiling. BMC Microbiol 2016;16:72.

25. Leonard RB, Mayer J, Sasser M, et al. Comparison of MIDI Sherlock system and pulsed-field gel electrophoresis in characterizing strains of methicillin-resistant *Staphylococcus aureus* from a recent hospital outbreak. J Clin Microbiol 1995; 33(10):2723.

26. Basu SS, McMinn MH, Giménez-Cassina Lopéz B, et al. Metal oxide laser ionization mass spectrometry imaging (MOLI MSI) using Cerium(IV) oxide. Anal Chem 2019;91(10):6800.

27. Cody RB, Laramée JA, Durst HD. Versatile new ion source for the analysis of materials in open air under ambient conditions. Anal Chem 2005;77(8):2297.

28. Pierce CY, Barr JR, Cody RB, et al. Ambient generation of fatty acid methyl ester ions from bacterial whole cells by direct analysis in real time (DART) mass spectrometry. Chem Commun (Camb) 2007;(8):807.

29. Cody RB, McAlpin CR, Cox CR, et al. Identification of bacteria by fatty acid profiling with direct analysis in real time mass spectrometry. Rapid Commun Mass Spectrom 2015;29(21):2007.

30. Cody RB. Saccharomyces cerevisiae and S. pastorianus species and strain differentiation by direct analysis in real time time-of-flight mass spectrometry. Rapid Commun Mass Spectrom 2020;34:e8835.

31. Phelps DL, Balog J, Gildea LF, et al. The surgical intelligent knife distinguishes normal, borderline and malignant gynaecological tissues using rapid evaporative ionisation mass spectrometry (REIMS). Br J Cancer 2018;118(10):1349.

32. Strittmatter N, Jones EA, Veselkov KA, et al. Analysis of intact bacteria using rapid evaporative ionisation mass spectrometry. Chem Commun (Camb) 2013; 49(55):6188.

33. Cameron SJ, Bolt F, Perdones-Montero A, et al. Rapid Evaporative Ionisation Mass Spectrometry (REIMS) provides accurate direct from culture species identification within the genus *Candida*. Sci Rep 2016;6:36788.

34. Bolt F, Cameron SJ, Karancsi T, et al. Automated high-throughput identification and characterization of clinically important bacteria and fungi using rapid evaporative ionization mass spectrometry. Anal Chem 2016;88(19):9419.

35. Pitt JJ. Principles and applications of liquid chromatography-mass spectrometry in clinical biochemistry. Clin Biochem Rev 2009;30(1):19.
36. Wolk DM, Kaleta EJ, Wysocki VH. PCR-electrospray ionization mass spectrometry: the potential to change infectious disease diagnostics in clinical and public health laboratories. J Mol Diagn 2012;14(4):295.
37. Strålin K, Rothman RE, Özenci V, et al. Performance of PCR/electrospray ionization-mass spectrometry on whole blood for detection of bloodstream microorganisms in patients with Suspected sepsis. J Clin Microbiol 2020;58:e01860.
38. Metzgar D, Frinder MW, Rothman RE, et al. The IRIDICA BAC BSI assay: rapid, sensitive and culture-independent identification of bacteria and *Candida* in Blood. PLoS One 2016;11(7):e0158186.
39. Jacob D, Sauer U, Housley R, et al. Rapid and high-throughput detection of highly pathogenic bacteria by Ibis PLEX-ID technology. PLoS One 2012;7(6):e39928.
40. Ifa DR, Wu C, Ouyang Z, et al. Desorption electrospray ionization and other ambient ionization methods: current progress and preview. Analyst 2010;135(4):669.
41. Meetani MA, Shin YS, Zhang S, et al. Desorption electrospray ionization mass spectrometry of intact bacteria. J Mass Spectrom 2007;42(9):1186.

Mass Cytometry, Imaging Mass Cytometry, and Multiplexed Ion Beam Imaging Use in a Clinical Setting

Raymond D. Devine, PhD, Gregory K. Behbehani, MD, PhD*

KEYWORDS

- Mass cytometry • Imaging mass cytometry • Multiplex ion beam imaging
- Mass spectroscopy time of flight • High-parameter data analysis

KEY POINTS

- Mass-tag–based antibody detection enables high-parameter analysis of cellular antigens by avoiding the spectral overlap that limits fluorescent-based antibody detection methods. Currently, this enables 40 to 60 parameter detection, but the theoretic limit is 100+ simultaneous measurement channels.
- Mass cytometry is used for measurement of cells in solution, whereas imaging mass cytometry and multiplexed ion beam imaging create high-parameter images of tissue sections.
- Each system can generate very high-dimensional data that are best analyzed with clustering or dimensionality reduction methods.
- These systems are ideal for characterizing complex cellular mixtures, or for monitoring functional processes at high resolution.

INTRODUCTION

Flow cytometry (FC) is a widely used tool in basic and clinical research with its ability to study malignancies, infectious diseases, and immune system function. Its utility is due to its ability, at a single-cell level, to detect any component recognized by an antibody. This utility, however, is constrained by the number of parameters that can be analyzed simultaneously. Most clinical flow cytometers can analyze between 4 and 15 parameters, this limitation is primarily due to fluorescent reporters and their spectral emission overlap. Recent advancements are overcoming this limitation such as multispectral flow cytometers that can recognize approximately 32 different parameters[1]; however, one of the most significant developments is mass cytometry (MC), and MC-based imaging.[2–7]

Division of Hematology, Department of Internal Medicine, The Ohio State University Wexner Medical Center, Comprehensive Cancer Center, Columbus, OH, USA
* Corresponding author. Division of Hematology, The Ohio State University and James Cancer Hospital, B305 Starling Loving Hall, 320 West 10th Avenue, Columbus, OH 43210.
E-mail address: Gregory.Behbehani@OSUMC.edu

Clin Lab Med 41 (2021) 297–308
https://doi.org/10.1016/j.cll.2021.03.008   labmed.theclinics.com

In principle, MC is similar to FC, as both use antibody-based detection at a single-cell level and generate similar data. The difference is that MC uses metal-tagged antibodies instead of fluorescently labeled antibodies. The cells, with the bound antibody-metal conjugates, are detected through time of flight mass spectrometry (TOF MS). TOF MS is able to distinguish ions of different atomic weights with less than 0.5% spillover into adjacent channels, yielding a high resolution that allows for a large increase in measurable parameters of the MC system. It is now considered routine to have panels of approximately 50 antibodies and up to 60 total measured ions, and this number is continuing to increase, with recent of additions of metals such as nanoparticle-tantalum–based antibody conjugation.[8] The theoretic upper limit of parameters is approximately 120 mass channels, which may be reached as the field continues to advance. Although MC has been a significant development, the application of metal-conjugated antibodies and TOF detection has continued to develop with imaging MC (IMC) and multiplexed ion beam imaging (MIBI).[4–6,9] IMC and MIBI both perform the same function of allowing very high-parameter detection of antibody binding to tissues, but the systems work in different ways. All 3 systems can enable very high-dimensional characterization of both surface antigens (to define cell identity), as well as intracellular antigens that can be used to characterize cellular functional properties.

MASS CYTOMETRY

MC, IMC, and MIBI have been talked about in the theoretic sense, and it is important to understand their specific operation. Generally, the procedure to stain cells for MC is similar to FC with some differences. The cells are incubated with antibodies as in FC; however, as a final step before processing, they must be incubated with a DNA intercalator or other stain to identify cells that were not antibody stained.[10] The samples run in pure water (or a very dilute organic salt solution) to avoid salt build up and signal loss in the instrument. This necessitates fixation of cells before running (to ensure that the antibodies remain attached). The diluted cell suspension is aerosolized, passing through the nebulizer and into a heating chamber to evaporate the water. The cells then pass into an induced argon plasma at a temperature of approximately 7000°K. The cells are completely vaporized, generating a cloud of positively charged ions. Uncharged atomic species and lower atomic mass (>75 Da) ions are filtered out. Due to the ionization, the resulting ions are almost all +1 and are thus accelerated with the same force, meaning lighter ions will accelerate faster and hit the detector earlier than the heavier ions. These ion strikes are then computationally processed into mass channel signals (based on the daily mass calibration of the machine). All of the ion measurements from the cloud formed by each cell are then integrated together, generating the data for the individual single-cell event that is exported as a Flow Cytometry Standard (FCS) file, which can be analyzed and processed like FC data (**Fig. 1**).

MC is particularly useful for the characterization of complex cell mixtures, or highly complex analyses of mixed cell populations. High-parameter analyses of malignant diseases, particularly leukemias, have been performed by several research groups.[11–16] These studies highlight the strength of high-parameter analysis: the ability to define rare cell types and characterize the functional properties of these cells. This has been used to identify rare immunophenotypic stem cell populations with low S-phase fractions in samples from patients with acute myeloid leukemia (AML) subtypes known to respond poorly to treatment. These slowly proliferating cells also had specific immunophenotypic markers that could potentially be targeted with

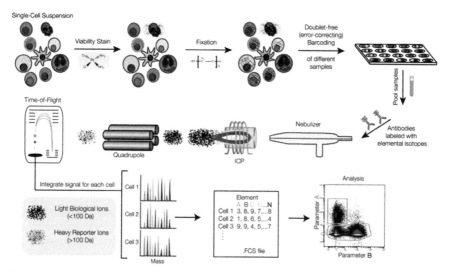

Fig. 1. An example of an MC workflow in which cells are stained for viability and also barcoded before being stained with antibodies. The cells are then nebulized into droplets before entering the mass cytometer. The cells are ionized into their individual isotopes and these ions are quantified by TOF MS. These ion strikes are integrated in a cell-by-cell basis resulting in single-cell measurements that are packaged into FCS files for downstream analysis. (*Adapted from* Spitzer MH, Nolan GP. Mass cytometry: single cells, many features. Cell. 2016;165(4):780–91; with permission.)

alternative therapies.[12] Ferrell and colleagues[13] used an MC approach to identify phenotypic changes that occur in the AML blast population in serial samples, whereas Fisher and colleagues[14] performed an analysis of bone marrow samples from patients with myelofibrosis and associated secondary AML to identify abnormal nuclear factor (NF)-κB pathway signaling in progenitor cell populations from patients with these diseases. Each of these assay approaches could eventually be harnessed to select therapeutic treatment strategies.

A major clinical application in which MC could prove useful is monitoring of immune system function. High-parameter assessment by MC allows the simultaneous assessment of a broad range of activation markers across a wide range of immune effector cells. This allows measurement of immune function and identification of novel immune cell subsets. Strauss-Albee and colleagues[17] mapped the diversity of NK cells across diverse donors to demonstrate relationships between viral exposure and NK diversity and differentiation. Another method developed by Newell and colleagues[18] combined MHC-tetramer staining with high-parameter surface immunophenotype assessment to the characterize a phenotypically distinct T-cell subset that was specific to the response against rotavirus infection. In the study of rheumatologic disease, Rao and colleagues[19] used MC to identify an expanded T-cell population that appears to drive B-cell activation in rheumatoid arthritis, and O'Gorman and colleagues[20] demonstrated distinct monocyte cytokine profiles associated with systemic lupus erythematous. These examples suggest that precise characterization aspects of immune function could be diagnostic in a variety of medical conditions.

High-parameter MC is also suited for assessment of immunotherapies because it enables characterization of malignant cells along with assessment of immune effector cells and how therapeutic interventions might alter their activation state. Showcasing the potential of MC for monitoring of cancer immunotherapy was recently performed in a mouse model.[21] In this study, MC was used to characterize a range of tissues from mice receiving either a successful immunotherapy or one known to be incapable of tumor rejection. This study showed successful immunotherapy response was associated with an expanded CD4 T-cell population systemically, rather than specifically in the tumor microenvironment. This suggests that human immunotherapy responses could be monitored systemically.[22,23] Clinically, the ability to make such assessments could enable the early detection of treatment resistance and allow for adaptive changes of therapeutic strategy.

IMAGING MASS CYTOMETRY

IMC is an immunocytochemistry (ICC) and immunohistochemistry (IHC) analog designed to use metal-labeled antibodies and an existing MC platform. Immunofluorescence analysis of fixed slide sections is limited to approximately 7 antibodies due to spectral overlap. Multiplex processing requires use of antibody stripping, dye bleaching, or other similar methods, which are labor-intensive and can cause antigen changes.[24] IMC system gets around this by using mass channels that can be detected without significant signal overlap, allowing simultaneous staining. The commercially available IMC system uses 2 connected instruments. The first performs laser ablation of the sample in 1-μm points and then transports the resulting ablated sample material into the second instrument, which is a standard MC platform. Tissue sections are cut at a 5-μm thickness before being dewaxed and rehydrated according to standard protocols.[25] The laser delivers a homogenized UV beam ($\lambda = 193$ nm) of 1-μm diameter, which is used to raster across the sample and ablate the antibody-stained tissue at a rate of 20 Hz. The ablation crater resulting from the laser is approximately 1 μm in diameter.[7] This ablated sample aerosol is then transported to the MC by helium gas flow, where it then enters the argon sheath gas of the standard MC. From there, the detection performs just like MC described previously, with each ablated point of the tissue being analyzed as would a single cell in solution. The resulting data is a 2-dimensional (2D) grid of 1-μm data points (pixels) that is outputted as a standard n-dimensional TIFF file (where there is a single monochromatic image for each measured parameter). To identify cellular and subcellular spaces, high-expression surface markers are included in the staining panel to assist in both cell identification and establishing cellular boundaries.

The high parametric nature of IMC data enables new insights into tissue biology, particularly in the study of cancerous tumors. Giesen and colleagues[6] showed that IMC was able to achieve subcellular resolution as well as traditional ICC/IHC methods. IMC analysis of fixed breast cancer tissue slides revealed unique cell population distributions among patients with otherwise similar tumor types, which would otherwise not be detectable using traditional methods. Work by Zhang and colleagues[26] used IMC analysis on slides of cancerous and paracancerous tissue and demonstrated a unique subpopulation of EpCAM$^+$ CD4$^+$ T cells infiltrating the tumor region. The use of a multiplex panel with IMC also showed these cells have dysfunctional phospho-p38, and MAP kinase signaling. These EpCAM$^+$ CD4$^+$ T cells also expressed PD-L1, CCR5, and CCR6, which would be expected to suppress the immune response.[26]

MULTIPLEXED ION BEAM IMAGING

Multiplexed ion beam imaging (MIBI) was developed simultaneously with early studies of MC in the Nolan laboratory and was first demonstrated in the 2014 publication by

Angelo and colleagues,[4] which demonstrated that it was possible to take formalin-fixed paraffin embedded (FFPE) breast tumor tissue sections and stain them with metal-conjugated antibodies. This allows for a generation of a 2D map of the tissue slide with markers already commonly used to diagnostic purposes but also novel markers in triple negative breast cancer samples. Originally a magnetic mass detection was used but current platforms use TOF analysis.[4,5] Staining protocols are similar to described previously in the IMC section. IMC and MIBI systems achieve their similar goals through different means. MIBI would be more appropriately called a secondary ion mass spectrometer (SIMS). SIMS, and by extension the MIBI, sputter the slide with a focused ion beam from an ion gun. The ion gun used in the MIBI is an oxygen duoplasmatron producing O− primary ions, and the sample is rasterized under the ion stream. This beam results in the ionization of the surface material and ejection of secondary ions. Once secondary ions are released, they pass through filters that remove common biological ions (eg, carbon, nitrogen). The ions that pass through the filters, are then accelerated for TOF analysis. Like in IMC, the data are exported as an n-dimensional TIFF file, which can subsequently be viewed as an image or segmented into individual cell events analyzed as FCS files. This allows analysis of the cell types present and how they relate to the tumor microenvironment architecture as a whole (**Fig. 2**).

Similar to IMC, the high-parameter measurement of tissue sections by MIBI allows for novel insights into tissue biology. Work by Keren and colleagues[5] demonstrated the utility of MIBI in understanding complex heterogenic environments of breast cancer tissue slides. For instance, they demonstrated that the tumor cells demonstrate a concentric pattern of myeloid derived suppressorlike cells, which are themselves surrounded by lymphocyte-rich regions.[5]

ADVANTAGES OF MASS-TAG DETECTION

Regardless of which system is used and for which purpose, there are several advantages and disadvantages of using heavy metal-conjugated antibodies or other heavy metal reagents and TOF MS detection.

- TOF mass detection allows for a high number a potential detection parameters (100+).
- Very low spillover between detection channels (<0.5%); however, not all mass species can be purified to 100% purity leading to isotopic contamination.
- Mass-tag measurements have wide dynamic ranges and are essentially free from background.
- Can be used to study cell manipulations that create autofluorescence that would otherwise be problematic for fluorescence-based detection methods.
- The mass cytometers only have a single detector for all channels, eliminating the complexity of adjusting and monitoring multiple detectors.
- Mass-tagged antibodies are currently made with metal chelating polymers that are very chemically stable.
- A variety of other heavy metal staining approaches can be used simultaneously with antibody-based antigen detection. This includes Iodo-deoxyuridine–based detection of DNA synthesis during S-phase,[27,28] cellular viability stains,[29] Te-based reagents for detection of cellular hypoxia,[30] and whole cell stains that can be used for cellular barcoding.[31,32]
- A variety of other chemical methods (eg, metal nanoparticles[33]) can be used to expand the number of useable mass channels and increase signal intensity.

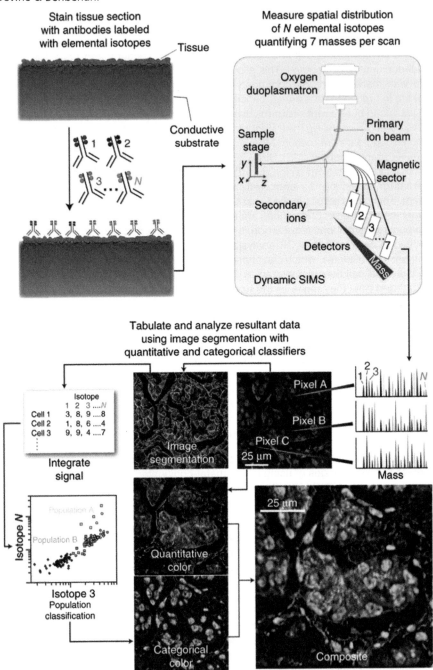

Fig. 2. An example workflow and result of MIBI in breast cancer tissue. Tissue sample slides are stained with metal conjugated antibodies before being loaded into a vacuum chamber. The sample surface is then rasterized with an ion beam to liberate the metal conjugated antibodies. Metal-conjugated antibodies are quantified with replicate scans of the same field of view. These are integrated into a composite image from a scanned slide and pseudocolored for the integrated ion signal. (*From* Angelo M, Bendall SC, Finck R, et al. Multiplexed ion beam imaging of human breast tumors. Nat Med. 2014;20(4):436–42; with permission.)

- Current reagents have relatively similar sensitivities across the mass range, but this sensitivity is lower than brighter fluorophores.

ADVANTAGES OF HIGH-PARAMETER CELLULAR CHARACTERIZATION

Although it is tempting to think that a sufficiently large number of low-parameter measurements could be combined to generate the same data that can be generated with MC approaches, there are a variety of applications that can be performed only if all parameters can be measured simultaneously. The simultaneous detection of a large number of parameters enables a variety of advantages:

- A large panel of surface markers can be used to model cellular differentiation and compare functional properties of cells across differentiation stages.
- Mass cytometric markers of cell cycle can be used in panels that measure complex functional properties and how they occur during each cell cycle stage.
- Use of cellular barcoding allows for the simultaneous staining and analysis (in the same tube) of several samples, thereby dramatically reducing technical variance between samples. Comparing normal and malignant cell samples in barcoded experiments can allow for detection of aberrant marker expression at very high resolution.
- Simultaneous measurement of several markers of cell phenotype in complex cell populations that can be identified only through the use of multiple markers.
- The interaction between complex cellular mixtures can be studied (in vitro cell killing assays, studies of the tumor microenvironment).

BIG DATA AND HIGH-DIMENSIONAL APPROACHES

As the systems listed previously can simultaneously measure approximately 50 channels, the data generated can be immense. A 42-antibody panel would require approximately 861 different biaxial plots to completely visualize the data. Fortunately, dimensionality reduction algorithms can deal with the complex single-cell data and organize it into more easily recognizable patterns. Metrics of cellular position and/or nearest cellular neighbor, can be incorporated into these high-dimensional analyses to capture special information in these analyses. Although there are many dimensionality reduction algorithms applicable to MC data, only a few are discussed here: spanning-tree analysis of density normalized events (SPADE), vi-stochastic neighbor embedding (vi-SNE), and Uniform Manifold Approximation and Projection (UMAP).

SPANNING-TREE ANALYSIS OF DENSITY NORMALIZED EVENTS

- SPADE was the first high-dimensional analysis technique commonly used for MC data.[34,35]
- SPADE begins with a pool of cell events drawn from all samples in the experiment.
- Analysis starts with a density-dependent down-sampling to maintain representation of rare cell populations.
- Agglomerative clustering is then performed by calculating the single-linkage distance between cells (across the user-specified clustering parameters) and grouping together the nearest neighbors iteratively until reaching the approximate prespecified number of clusters.
- These clusters then become nodes of a minimum spanning tree, with the nodes linked to one another based on their median expression of the clustering markers.

- The spanning tree result is then re-created for each individual sample by adding each cell event to the node of the common tree that is most similar to it. This creates nodes that are greatly expanded or absent in sample-specific patterns. The trees can be interacted with by the user in a GUI environment, which enables manual identification of the cell types based on the median expression of markers.
- Advantages of SPADE
  - Because clusters are generated using all cells in the experiment, it creates similar clusters across each sample allowing for "apples-to-apples" comparisons between different samples. This is particularly useful for rapidly calculating parameters like fold change and population density changes
  - The density-dependent down-sampling ensures representation of rare cell populations
- Disadvantages of SPADE
  - The minimum spanning tree's global structure is random, and does not necessarily reflect the global structure of the underlying data. Each time the analysis is run a different common tree structure will be created.
  - By nature, the clustering groups cells together, interrupting any continuous variance. This makes it difficult to use SPADE for analyzing progressions from 1 cell type or cell state to another.
- In retrospective analyses, SPADE has been demonstrated to predict human immunodeficiency virus outcomes,[36] analyze aberrant monocytic subsets in chronic myelocytic leukemia,[37] demonstrate how cell cycle state interacts with treatment responses,[12] and identified T-cell populations that can predict graft versus host disease.[38]
- SPADE has been used in conjunction with IMC technology to study FFPE samples of breast cancer samples demonstrating unique marker distribution patterns among samples that were determined to be of the same type of breast cancer.[6]

T-DISTRIBUTED STOCHASTIC NEIGHBOR EMBEDDING/VI-DISTRIBUTED STOCHASTIC NEIGHBOR EMBEDDING AND UNIFORM MANIFOLD APPROXIMATION AND PROJECTION

- vi-SNE is an adaption of t-distributed Stochastic Neighbor Embedding approach (t-SNE) specific for cytometry data analysis.[39]
- UMAP stands for Uniform Manifold Approximation and Projection and was developed primarily as an improvement on t-SNE to better preserve global data structure and improve run-time performance.[40]
- Both approaches seek to approximate the overall data structure, and key to both is the utilization of a stochastic gradient descent optimization step that iteratively modifies the final data projection to make it best represent the underlying high-dimensional data.
- This final step helps to ensure that the data representation is not overly influenced by a single data parameter or by large changes that occur during a progression in the data set.
- The most common output from both analyses is a 2D scatter plot of individual cell events (although both algorithms can create higher-dimensional representations). These plots look similar to PCA plots, but do not have the underlying linearity found in PCA. After the analysis, in both cases, each cell event is assigned 2 or more new parameters that define its place in this representation (for instance t-SNE1 and t-SNE2 or UMAP1 and UMAP2).

- A thorough descriptions of the differences between t-SNE and UMAP is beyond the scope of this article, but some of the key difference are discussed in detail in the original UMAP publication.[40]
- Advantages of t-SNE and UMAP
  - Especially useful for progressive changes that occur as a biological response or cell development and differentiation. Vi-SNE is most commonly used to perform analysis of broad cellular systems to discern global changes in individual cells leading to discovery of novel cell subtypes.[12,17,19,23,35,41]
  - All analyzed cells are individually represented in the final data projection and each cell has an essentially unique position in the projection.
  - The global data structure represents all samples, allowing individual samples to have sample-specific versions of the data projection.
- Disadvantages of t-SNE and UMAP
  - A major drawback of the t-SNE and UMAP techniques stems from one of their primary advantages; they place each single cell into an essentially unique position relative to other cells in the experiment, which makes objectively comparing similar cell subpopulations across samples much more difficult. A reference point can be created by including some type of "normal" reference sample in the experiment, however, abnormal cell events will never perfectly overlap with the normal reference populations.
  - Both t-SNE and UMAP projections are heavily influence by the abundance of cells in the experiment; this creates large areas of the final data projections specific for high abundance cell types even if these have relatively little meaningful biologic variation, as a result, the properties of rare cell populations can become more difficult to discern.
  - For computational reasons, both approaches are commonly used only on a sampling of cell events from the experiment, further reducing the utility of the methods for rare cell detection.
- t-SNE/vi-SNE would have been most useful in instances in which there are progressive biological changes of interest, or for identification of rare cells that are very phenotypically unique.
  - vi-SNE has been used for MRD tracking in AML and acute lymphocytic leukemia, and also been used to track abnormal progenitor cells in AML induction. Vi-SNE may also be applicable in instances of differentiation therapy in hematological malignancies.[5,11,13]

CLINICS CARE POINTS

- MC, IMC, and MIBI are capable of a highly parametric analysis of highly complex cell populations or biologic processes.

- These methods have most commonly been applied to the study of the immune system, cancer cells, or the intersection of the two in investigations of cancer immunotherapy.

- MC is now a relatively mature technology and both IMC and MIBI are maturing rapidly. All are currently being used in clinical research studies. All 3 technologies could potentially be adapted for use in clinical care.

- All are best suited to the study of relatively rare cell types that require the use of several markers for identification or characterization, particularly if the cells of interest are present in a complex mixture.

- Because of the small spillover of the TOF analysis and importantly, the small isotopic impurities in the metal-tagged reagents, it remains important to consider the design of the staining panel. Avoid having low-abundance antigens in channels that will receive spillover from higher-abundance channels. Compensation is possible, but significantly more complicated than FC compensation.[42,43]

- All 3 systems are highly complex and require dedicated and highly trained operators, as well as specialized computer hardware, ventilation, gas supplies, power supply, and isolation from vibration. Each system is dependent on ongoing maintenance and calibration and will generally require contracted service support from the manufacturer.

- Due to the large amount of data generated, meaningful analysis of experiments performed using these systems typically requires experience with a variety of dimensionality reduction approaches.

- Although very complex, once a panel and workflow are optimized, a new sample can run relatively rapidly in approximately 2 to 5 days. This makes these techniques useful for developing data that could be used in the timeframe of clinical decision making.

SUMMARY

Research and clinical communities continue to develop a greater appreciation of the immense complexity of neoplastic diseases and the intricacies of immune system regulation. With these areas becoming central to newer targeted and personalized therapeutic interventions, particularly within the fields of immunotherapies and cellular therapies, the greater understanding of the many different normal and abnormal cell types and regulatory molecules central to these new treatment approaches has led to the need for much more advanced cytometric measurement technologies. Mass spectrometry-based cytometry (MC, IMC, and MIBI) technologies are uniquely well suited to these research and clinical investigations. The data generated by these technologies is also very complementary to next-generation bulk and single-cell sequencing approaches. High-parameter data generated in such analyses enables novel computational analysis approaches that have generated new insights into immune and cancer cell function. These approaches will greatly enhance our understanding of the immune system, neoplastic diseases, and can be used to develop new therapies and personalize them for the patients who will benefit the most from them.

ACKNOWLEDGEMENTS

This work was supported by the Pelotonia Fellowship Program. Any opinions, findings, and conclusions expressed in this material are those of the author(s) and do not necessarily reflect those of the Pelotonia Fellowship Program.

DISCLOSURE

The authors declare they have no conflict of interests.

REFERENCES

1. Feher K, von Volkmann K, Kirsch J, et al. Multispectral flow cytometry: the consequences of increased light collection. Cytometry A 2016;89(7):681–9.
2. Spitzer MH, Nolan GP. Mass cytometry: single cells, many features. Cell 2016; 165(4):780–91.
3. Tanner SD, Baranov VI, Ornatsky OI, et al. An introduction to mass cytometry: fundamentals and applications. Cancer Immunol Immunother 2013;62(5):955–65.
4. Angelo M, Bendall SC, Finck R, et al. Multiplexed ion beam imaging of human breast tumors. Nat Med 2014;20(4):436–42.

5. Keren L, Bosse M, Thompson S, et al. MIBI-TOF: a multiplexed imaging platform relates cellular phenotypes and tissue structure. Sci Adv 2019;5(10):eaax5851.

6. Giesen C, Wang HAO, Schapiro D, et al. Highly multiplexed imaging of tumor tissues with subcellular resolution by mass cytometry. Nat Methods 2014;11(4): 417–+.

7. Wang HAO, Grolimund D, Giesen C, et al. Fast chemical imaging at high spatial resolution by laser ablation inductively coupled plasma mass spectrometry. Anal Chem 2013;85(21):10107–16.

8. Zhang Y, Zabinyakov N, Majonis D, et al. Tantalum oxide nanoparticle-based mass tag for mass cytometry. Anal Chem 2020;92(8):5741–9.

9. Bodenmiller B. Multiplexed epitope-based tissue imaging for discovery and healthcare applications. Cell Syst 2016;2(4):225–38.

10. Behbehani GK. Immunophenotyping by mass cytometry. Methods Mol Biol 2019; 2032:31–51.

11. Amir el AD, Davis KL, Tadmor MD, et al. viSNE enables visualization of high dimensional single-cell data and reveals phenotypic heterogeneity of leukemia. Nat Biotechnol 2013;31(6):545–52.

12. Behbehani GK, Samusik N, Bjornson ZB, et al. Mass cytometric functional profiling of acute myeloid leukemia defines cell-cycle and immunophenotypic properties that correlate with known responses to therapy. Cancer Discov 2015;5(9):988–1003.

13. Ferrell PB Jr, Diggins KE, Polikowsky HG, et al. High-dimensional analysis of acute myeloid leukemia reveals phenotypic changes in persistent cells during induction therapy. PLoS One 2016;11(4):e0153207.

14. Fisher DAC, Malkova O, Engle EK, et al. Mass cytometry analysis reveals hyperactive NF Kappa B signaling in myelofibrosis and secondary acute myeloid leukemia. Leukemia 2017;31(9):1962–74.

15. Levine JH, Simonds EF, Bendall SC, et al. Data-driven phenotypic dissection of AML reveals progenitor-like cells that correlate with prognosis. Cell 2015; 162(1):184–97.

16. Behbehani GK, Finck R, Samusik N, et al. Profiling myelodysplastic syndromes by mass cytometry demonstrates abnormal progenitor cell phenotype and differentiation. Cytometry B Clin Cytom 2020;98(2):131–45.

17. Strauss-Albee DM, Fukuyama J, Liang EC, et al. Human NK cell repertoire diversity reflects immune experience and correlates with viral susceptibility. Sci Transl Med 2015;7(297):297ra115.

18. Newell EW, Sigal N, Nair N, et al. Combinatorial tetramer staining and mass cytometry analysis facilitate T-cell epitope mapping and characterization. Nat Biotechnol 2013;31(7):623–9.

19. Rao DA, Gurish MF, Marshall JL, et al. Pathologically expanded peripheral T helper cell subset drives B cells in rheumatoid arthritis. Nature 2017;542(7639):110–4.

20. O'Gorman WE, Kong DS, Balboni IM, et al. Mass cytometry identifies a distinct monocyte cytokine signature shared by clinically heterogeneous pediatric SLE patients. J Autoimmun 2017. https://doi.org/10.1016/j.jaut.2017.03.010.

21. Spitzer MH, Carmi Y, Reticker-Flynn NE, et al. Systemic immunity is required for effective cancer immunotherapy. Cell 2017;168(3):487–502 e15.

22. Wistuba-Hamprecht K, Martens A, Weide B, et al. Establishing high dimensional immune signatures from peripheral blood via mass cytometry in a discovery cohort of stage IV melanoma patients. J Immunol 2017;198(2):927.

23. Romee R, Rosario M, Berrien-Elliott MM, et al. Cytokine-induced memory-like natural killer cells exhibit enhanced responses against myeloid leukemia. 10.1126/scitranslmed.aaf2341. Sci Transl Med 2016;8(357). 357ra123.
24. Narhi LO, Caughey DJ, Horan T, et al. Effect of three elution buffers on the recovery and structure of monoclonal antibodies. Anal Biochem 1997;253(2):236–45.
25. Robertson D, Savage K, Reis-Filho JS, et al. Multiple immunofluorescence labelling of formalin-fixed paraffin-embedded (FFPE) tissue. BMC Cell Biol 2008;9:13.
26. Zhang T, Lv JW, Tan ZY, et al. Immunocyte profiling using single-cell mass cytometry reveals EpCAM(+) CD4(+) T cells abnormal in colon cancer. Front Immunol 2019. https://doi.org/10.3389/fimmu.2019.01571.
27. Behbehani GK. Mass cytometric cell cycle analysis. Methods Mol Biol 2019;1989:193–215.
28. Behbehani GK, Bendall SC, Clutter MR, et al. Single-cell mass cytometry adapted to measurements of the cell cycle. Cytometry A 2012;81(7):552–66.
29. Fienberg HG, Simonds EF, Fantl WJ, et al. A platinum-based covalent viability reagent for single-cell mass cytometry. Cytometry A 2012;81a(6):467–75.
30. Edgar LJ, Vellanki RN, Halupa A, et al. Identification of hypoxic cells using an organotellurium tag compatible with mass cytometry. Angew Chem Int Edit 2014;53(43):11473–7.
31. Behbehani GK, Thom C, Zunder ER, et al. Transient partial permeabilization with saponin enables cellular barcoding prior to surface marker staining. Cytometry A 2014;85(12):1011–9.
32. Zunder ER, Finck R, Behbehani GK, et al. Palladium-based mass tag cell barcoding with a doublet-filtering scheme and single-cell deconvolution algorithm. Nat Protoc 2015;10(2):316–33.
33. Schulz AR, Stanislawiak S, Baumgart S, et al. Silver nanoparticles for the detection of cell surface antigens in mass cytometry. Cytometry A 2017;91(1):25–33.
34. Qiu P, Simonds EF, Bendall SC, et al. Extracting a cellular hierarchy from high-dimensional cytometry data with SPADE. Nat Biotechnol 2011;29(10):886–91.
35. Bendall SC, Simonds EF, Qiu P, et al. Single-cell mass cytometry of differential immune and drug responses across a human hematopoietic continuum. Science 2011;332(6030):687–96.
36. Aghaeepour N, Chattopadhyay P, Chikina M, et al. A benchmark for evaluation of algorithms for identification of cellular correlates of clinical outcomes. Cytometry A 2016;89(1):16–21.
37. Selimoglu-Buet D, Wagner-Ballon O, Saada V, et al. Characteristic repartition of monocyte subsets as a diagnostic signature of chronic myelomonocytic leukemia. Blood 2015;125(23):3618–26.
38. Kim BS, Nishikii H, Baker J, et al. Treatment with agonistic DR3 antibody results in expansion of donor Tregs and reduced graft-versus-host disease. Blood 2015;126(4):546–57.
39. van der Maaten L, Hinton G. Visualizing data using t-SNE. J Mach Learn Res 2008;9:2579–605.
40. Melville J, McInnes L, Healy J. UMAP: uniform manifold approximation and projection for dimension reduction. arXiv 2018.
41. Ribas A, Shin DS, Zaretsky J, et al. PD-1 blockade expands intratumoral memory T cells. Cancer Immunol Res 2016;4(3):194–203.
42. Chevrier S, Crowell HL, Zanotelli VRT, et al. Compensation of signal spillover in suspension and imaging mass cytometry. Cell Syst 2018;6(5):612–620 e5.
43. Sekhri P, Kim MY, Behbehani GK. Unlabeled competitor antibody to reduce nonlinear signal spillover in mass cytometry. Cytometry A 2019;95(8):898–909.

Bringing Matrix-Assisted Laser Desorption/Ionization Mass Spectrometry Imaging to the Clinics

Sankha S. Basu, MD, PhD[a], Nathalie Y.R. Agar, PhD[b,c,d],*

KEYWORDS

- Mass spectrometry imaging • MALDI • Cancer • Infectious disease
- Drug distribution • Clinical

KEY POINTS

- Matrix-assisted laser desorption/ionization (MALDI) mass spectrometry imaging (MSI) represents a powerful analytical platform for clinical tissue diagnostics.
- MALDI MSI has been moving from the basic research to the translational and clinical space.
- Clinical implementation of MALDI MSI requires consideration of the diagnostic question being addressed, clinical workflows and specimens, as well as the strengths and limitations of different platforms.

INTRODUCTION

Mass spectrometry imaging (MSI) is an emerging set of analytical techniques that hold promise in changing pathology and tissue-based diagnostics.[1] In its simplest sense, MSI is an analytical chemistry application in which a target is analyzed using a mass spectrometer in at least 2 spatial dimensions and, in doing so, preserves the relative spatial location of molecules during analysis. The net effect is the creation of a biochemical map or ion image, or, more precisely, hundreds to thousands of concomitant ion images, each of which corresponds to the spatial distribution of a particular ion. In clinical applications, MSI can be used to map both endogenous and exogenous small molecules,[2] lipids,[3] as well as peptides and proteins,[4] depending on the ionization technique and mass analyzer used. Several ionization techniques have been described, including secondary ionization mass spectrometry (SIMS) and

[a] Department of Pathology, Brigham and Women's Hospital, Harvard Medical School, Boston, MA 02115, USA; [b] Department of Neurosurgery, Brigham and Women's Hospital, Harvard Medical School, Boston, MA 02115, USA; [c] Department of Radiology, Brigham and Women's Hospital, Harvard Medical School, Boston, MA, USA; [d] Department of Cancer Biology, Dana-Farber Cancer Institute, Harvard Medical School, Boston, MA 02115, USA
* Corresponding author.
E-mail address: Nathalie_Agar@dfci.harvard.edu

Clin Lab Med 41 (2021) 309–324
https://doi.org/10.1016/j.cll.2021.03.009
0272-2712/21/© 2021 Elsevier Inc. All rights reserved.
labmed.theclinics.com

ambient electrospray ionization such as desorption electrospray ionization (DESI), although these are outside of the scope of the review and are reviewed elsewhere.[5] This article focuses on MSI applications that use matrix-assisted laser ionization/desorption (MALDI) as the ionization source.

Although there are many variations in sample preparation and analysis in MALDI MSI, the overall approach is generally similar. MALDI MSI begins with mounting a specimen, such as a cryosectioned tissue, onto a conductive slide or plate. A chemical matrix, commonly a small organic acid such as α-cyano-4-hydroxycinnamic acid (α-CHCA) or 2,5-dihydroxybenzoic acid (DHB), is applied to the surface either through spotting or spraying a solvent containing that matrix or by subliming the matrix onto the specimen. The matrix is then dried, the sample is moved to the source and placed under vacuum, and a region of interest is selected for analysis. Analysis is performed by firing a laser at the surface that desorbs ions from the tissue, which are then analyzed by the mass spectrometer. The most common mass spectrometers used in MALDI MSI are time of flight (TOF) mass analyzers. For certain applications, high-resolution mass spectrometers such as Fourier transform ion cyclotron resonance (FT-ICR) MS provide more robust and specific analysis. More recently, ion mobility has been added to these instruments to enhance their analytical power. Although MALDI MSI was described more than 20 years ago,[6] it is in the last few years that significant inroads into the translational and clinical space were made. This article provides a brief overview on clinical workflows; reviews clinical opportunities to use MALDI MSI, such as neoplastic and infectious diseases; and reviews some analytical parameters to consider when thinking about these applications.

CLINICAL WORKFLOWS AND OPPORTUNITIES

Before discussing MALDI MSI applications, it is valuable to provide the setting and clinical workflows in which these different applications can be used. There are no universal clinical settings, because there are differences between smaller community hospitals, academic centers, and private practices as well as regional and international differences. However, this is discussed in a general sense, with additional details as pertains to our own setting working in an academic medical center. In a broad sense, most clinical specimens are analyzed by pathologists in either clinical pathology (CP) or anatomic pathology (AP). AP largely consists of analysis of tissue specimens, and is often subdivided into surgical pathology, cytopathology, and autopsy pathology, and can be further divided into subspecialized areas focused on different tissues or organs. AP covers almost all clinical tissue specimens and is therefore the primary area for MSI-based approaches. In contrast, CP, also known as laboratory medicine, largely involves the analysis of liquid specimens, such as blood, urine, cerebrospinal fluid, and other body fluids, and is further divided into chemistry, hematology, microbiology, molecular pathology, and blood banking/transfusion medicine. There are tissue specimens such as lymph nodes and bone marrow biopsies that are handled by hematopathologists and other areas of overlap. For simplicity, the focus in this review is on areas traditionally overseen in AP.

Most tissue specimens are obtained through surgical excisions or biopsies in the operating room or through certain outpatient procedures such as colonoscopies. In certain cases, the surgeon collects a small representative section for intraoperative analysis, or the so-called frozen section procedure,[7] in which a tissue sample is brought to the pathology frozen section room, where it is rapidly frozen in an embedding medium, sectioned using a cryotome, mounted on a glass slide, and quickly stained with hematoxylin-eosin (H&E). A pathologist then performs microscopic analysis and provides an impression to the surgeon. Common questions include whether tumor cells are present at a surgical margin, whether any lesional tissue is consistent with an infectious or neoplastic process, and, in the latter case, whether it contains benign or malignant cells. One of the key advantages of frozen section, and microscopic examination in general, is the ability to preserve spatial variations in the tissue. This ability is particularly important in processes such as cancer or infections that can be heterogenous or require high spatial resolution. However, there are limitations such as the turnaround time, some distortion or artifact that comes from freezing, as well as variability in the pathologic interpretation, particularly when it comes to difficult or borderline cases. Also, this technique is largely limited to H&E staining, which, although extremely valuable, cannot provide molecular, protein, or biochemical characterization, which are critical features of these disease processes. Many further details, such as tumor classification, aggressiveness, or the presence or absence of specific genomic alterations, are deferred to the evaluation of permanent section.

Permanent sections constitute a much larger fraction of pathologic specimens. To create a permanent section, the specimen is fixed in formalin, cut into representative sections, processed through a series of washing and preservation steps, and then embedded in paraffin wax. These formalin-fixed paraffin-embedded (FFPE) tissues are then cut using a microtome, mounted onto a glass slide, where the pathologist can perform a more detailed histologic analysis, which may include special stains, most notably immunohistochemical stains to determine the presence or absence of a specific protein, receptor, or other biomarker. Additional special stains are also available, including Gram, silver, acid-fast, mucicarmine, as well as many other stains that can help to detect specific pathogen types in the case of an infection being suspected. Although these FFPE specimens provide a much larger arsenal of tools, they come at the cost of time compared with frozen section, because these can take time to generate, stain, and then analyze on the order of days rather than minutes or hours. There are other areas, such as cytopathology, where fluids or cells collected by fine-needle aspiration or other means are still reviewed by pathologists using similar approaches either directly or after being preserved and reviewed as slides from cell blocks.

CLINICAL DIAGNOSTIC APPLICATIONS
Cancer Diagnostics

Cancer often leads the way in new treatment and diagnostic approaches. MSI is no exception, because many publications related to clinical MSI are cancer related. Although much of the development and optimization of MALDI MSI has been done on animal tissues, the past decade has seen a growing number of MALDI MSI studies using clinical samples. Many of these studies include FFPE or tissue microarray specimens because these tend to be the most abundantly available clinical tissues, although some have analyzed fresh or frozen tissues. Studies have included a wide variety of cancers, including, but not limited to, lung,[8–10] breast,[11–15] gastrointestinal,[8,16–22] genitourinary,[23–28] gynecologic,[29–32] renal,[33,34] and brain.[35–38] Rather than reviewing work done on each cancer type and subtype, this article discusses more global considerations and highlights specific examples where pertinent.

Tumor identification and subsequent classification remain among the primary roles of the pathologist. This process may involve identifying the presence of malignancy at frozen section or providing more detailed classification on permanent sections. The primary modalities of tumor classification involve morphologic analysis of H&E-stained sections combined with immunohistochemistry of characteristic biomarkers, although genetic and genomic characterization have a growing role.[39] Still, each of these modalities can be time, labor, and cost intensive. In addition, there remain some gray areas or borderline cases where conventional approaches struggle to differentiate these entities and, to address these, there has been an active effort to use newer approaches such as MALDI MSI. One recent example by McDowell and colleagues[40] used MALDI MSI on FFPE specimens to differentiate pancreatic ductal adenocarcinomas based on differences in the N-glycosidase–released N-linked glycome. Gleason scoring for prostate cancer is another area where there remains diagnostically challenging cases, and Randall and colleagues[23] used MALDI MSI to characterize tumors from different Gleason grade tumors, which showed very different metabolic profiles. In another example, Calligaris and colleagues[36] used MALDI MSI on frozen samples to differentiate pituitary adenomas in as little as 30 minutes by imaging the hormone secreted by the cell of origin.

Tumor staging represents another critical element in cancer diagnostics, because focal tumors can potentially be cured by surgical resection alone, whereas cancers that have spread to lymph nodes or more distant metastatic sites generally require more aggressive or systemic treatments such as chemotherapy or radiation. Imaging modalities such as PET computed tomography or MRI can help with staging but cannot detect small numbers of cells in lymph nodes, which would change the tumor stage. Some surgical resections contain numerous lymph nodes, and currently each lymph node must be carefully reviewed by a pathologist to detect metastases and a few malignant cells could be missed. If a different modality, such as MSI, could improve sensitivity or reduce the time needed for analysis, this could help both patients as well as diagnosticians. The potential to use lipidomic signatures to detect lymph node metastases has been demonstrated for breast and thyroid tumors using DESI MSI,[41] and it stands to reason a similar approach could be used for MALDI MSI. Using a different approach, Mittal and colleagues[42] performed MALDI MSI on primary endometrial tumors and found that the likelihood to metastasize could be predicted accurately (88% tumors correctly classified) without having to look at the lymph nodes themselves. Although using such a predictive approach would be unconventional, it highlights a potential future avenue for MALDI MSI to prognosticate metastasis.

Because of its curative potential, surgical resection remains the treatment of choice for many focal tumors. Carefully determining the extent of tumor invasion is key to determining local spread. Conventional approaches use either frozen section for intraoperative guidance or assessment on permanent section to determine whether there remains any tumor at the margins of the cancer. One of the more exciting clinical MS applications is MS in the operating room as a tool for surgical guidance. By monitoring the chemical signature of the tissue, the mass spectrometer can provide faster and potentially more sensitive and accurate tumor detection. Much of the intraoperative MS work has focused on ambient MS methods because it was once thought that MALDI MSI could not be done fast enough. However, the authors have shown that it can be done in as little as 3 to 5 minutes,[43] on par with the time it takes for frozen section. Although this is not as fast as some of the intraoperative ambient approaches,[44–46] it allows clinicians to systematically cover larger areas and provides higher spatial resolution, which may be important in very heterogenous tumors or those with micrometastases.

Drug Distribution

For cancer treatment, not only are effective drugs needed but they are needed in the target tissues at appropriate concentrations. Liquid chromatography–tandem MS (LC-MS/MS) has seen increasing use in clinical chemistry laboratories, most notably in toxicology and therapeutic drug monitoring. For most drugs, there is a good correlation between circulating levels and clinical efficacy. However, for other drugs, the level in the blood may not correlate with the level in the target tissue of interest for several reasons, including host metabolism, pharmacokinetics, pharmacogenomics, and perfusion and vascularization of tissue. Subtherapeutic levels could lead to ineffective treatment as well as an environment suitable for clonal evolution and development of drug resistance. Conventionally, to determine tissue drug levels, the tissue would be weighed, homogenized, and the drug extracted before analysis. Standard curves would be performed by spiking normal tissue. Although such an approach is more widely used and vetted, homogenizing tissue leads to loss of spatial distribution of the drug. Another issue is best highlighted by a RAF inhibitor trial where the drug was shown to be effective in a murine flank model but not against intracranial implanted tumors, and the blood-brain barrier was hypothesized to be the cause.[47] Interestingly, the relative penetration of drug seemed to be adequate in both the brain and the flank. However, high-spatial-resolution MALDI MSI showed that, although the drug was perfusing the tumor, it was not diffusing into the tumor parenchyma because of thickened and abnormal vessels within the tumor, highlighting the importance of characterizing intratumor drug distribution. Additional literature reviewing progress in drug distribution by MALDI MSI can be found elsewhere.[48–50]

Infectious Disease Diagnostics

Before discussing MSI applications for infectious disease diagnostics, it is worth considering the major classes of human pathogens, namely viruses, bacteria, fungi, and parasites. Unlike cancer, where cancer cells largely share the same biochemical and metabolic pathways as other cells in the body, albeit commonly at nonphysiologic levels, most pathogens harbor distinct biochemical pathways producing distinct biomolecules, not generally produced by humans. The ability to leverage these differences based on their unique mass-to-charge ratios makes MS a powerful and agnostic method to detect pathogens in clinical specimens. Various applications to detect different classes of organisms are discussed here.

Viruses have had an outsized impact in humans over the past few decades, including annual pandemics such as influenza and emerging viruses such as Ebola, Zika, and severe acute respiratory syndrome coronavirus-2 (SARS-CoV-2). When it comes to MS, the ability to uniquely distinguish pathogens relies on distinguishing the pathogens from background molecules. Because viruses do not generally have their own unique biochemical or metabolic pathways, detection of viral proteins is the most reliable and logical approach to detecting these in tissue. In most cases, viruses are detected using polymerase chain reaction (PCR)–based approaches, and the presence or absence of a virus is generally enough to guide diagnosis and management. However, there are several scenarios where tissue imaging may provide an additional benefit. One example is in neurologic infections, where inclusion bodies are seen in the tissue. Immunohistochemical staining may provide nonspecific binding with nonviral proteins leading to false-positivity. In contrast, formalin fixation and paraffin embedding may lead to damage to the DNA or RNA, resulting in poor PCR amplification in broad-range sequencing or allele-specific PCRs. Despite MALDI MSI being available for some time, there is limited evidence of detection of viral proteins in tissue. However, it has been shown that virus-infected tissues may show different metabolic and proteomic patterns, which may help identify biomarkers of infection.[51]

Bacteria are perhaps the most ubiquitous microorganisms in both the external and internal human environments, and the proper identification and distinguishing of both commensal and pathogenic bacterial infections is critical in many patients. Although bacterial culture remains the gold standard of bacterial detection, identification, and phenotypic testing, there are several challenges that arise in the diagnostic setting. First, patients are often treated with antibiotics and, as a result, many of the organisms do not survive culture. Also, there are organisms that do not survive the preanalytical and processing steps and therefore do not grow in culture, although there may be evidence of suppurative inflammation or organisms revealed by Gram stain in tissue. Even then, it might take several days to perform these special stains. The ability to detect bacteria based on microbial signatures or specific bacterial metabolites would be of great value in the clinical setting. One example of using such an approach is presented by Juříková and colleagues,[52] where they used a rat model of *Pseudomonas aeruginosa* infection to show the presence in the lung of pyoverdine, a characteristic fluorescent siderophore and virulence factor commonly expressed in these organisms. In another approach similar to MALDI, called metal oxide laser ionization (MOLI) MS, cerium oxide can be used as the matrix to reveal unique bacterial fatty acids with the same US Food and Drug Administration (FDA)–approved MALDI-TOF MS instruments currently available in many clinical microbiology laboratories.[53] By applying this using an MSI approach in a proof-of-concept pseudoinfection model, extracted and spotted bacterial lipids were shown to be distinguishable from mouse brain lipids.[54]

Among bacteria, mycobacteria pose a particular challenge in pathology, due in part to their low organism burden in disease. For example, *Mycobacterium tuberculosis*, perhaps the most widespread infection worldwide, is particularly difficult to detect in tissue. Despite a wide area of granulomatous inflammation, often only a few organisms are detectable in tissue. For this reason, new and rapid techniques in mycobacterial detection and diagnosis in tissue specimens are helpful. Like other bacteria, mycobacterial organisms have unique biochemical products, most notably mycolic acids. Mycolic acid is not a single molecule but a group of long-chain fatty acids, which can exceed 100 carbons in length, which form a waxy membrane. This waxy membrane provides the acid-fastness, and hence their name acid-fast bacilli. High-performance liquid chromatography (HPLC) analysis of mycolic acids was once commonly used to classify different mycobacterial species, but this has largely been replaced with nucleic acid–based, or more recently MALDI-TOF–based, identification. Although MALDI-TOF classification can be used on mycobacterial isolates, there are limited studies using MSI to detect mycobacteria in tissue. One recent study by Blanc and colleagues[55] showed, in mouse and rabbit mycobacterial infection models, the presence of phosphatidyl-myo-inositol mannoside and phosphoinositol-tuberculostearic acid, which are mycobacteria-specific lipids, in the lungs of these animals. Even more importantly, the same group showed that certain antituberculosis drugs, such as moxifloxacin, fail to penetrate the necrotizing granulomas, suggestive of potential windows or niches where the organism may survive or even evolve at subtherapeutic drug concentration.[56]

Fungi are another important class of organisms where MSI approaches may provide significant benefit. Infectious fungal pathogens, such as yeast, molds, and dimorphic molds, are a growing problem in the clinical arena, most notably in immunocompromised hosts. With the increased use of hematopoietic stem cell transplants and expansion of cellular therapies such as chimeric antigen receptor T-cell therapies, which promise to turn the tide on several hematopoietic and solid organ malignancies, the prevalence of fungal morbidity and mortality has continued to increase as more patients experience significant immunosuppression. In the context of tissue-based microbial diagnostics, there are a few aspects of fungal infections that are important to note compared with bacterial and mycobacterial disease. For one, both the relative size of fungi and their relative burden may be considerably greater than in bacterial and especially mycobacterial disease. Even the smallest yeast can be 10 to 20 times larger than bacteria. In addition, in most cases of fungal infection, the organism is apparent on histology. As such, high spatial resolution may be less of a concern. Some of the specific and commonly encountered applications include lung wedge resections, which present with evidence of fungal forms and fungal sinusitis. In both cases, the more commonly encountered organisms include *Aspergillus* species and *Mucorales* species, such as *Mucor* or *Rhizopus*. Although there are morphologic features that can distinguish these organisms, often these require more extensive special stains, such as silver staining, which can delay diagnosis. Also, the longer the organism resides in the tissue, the more atypical its histologic features can become. Therefore, the ability to use chemical signatures to distinguish these organisms may be of significant utility. Also, the speed at which this could be done would be significantly faster than nucleic acid sequencing–based approaches, which can take several days or longer, particularly because most of these must be performed at specialty reference laboratories. There is ample literature showing the ability to differentiate molds by MALDI,[57,58] so these could be applied to these tissues as well. Although there are limited applications for diagnosis of infections in human tissues, *Aspergillus* siderophores ferricrocin and triacetylfusarinine C were detected in a rat model of *Aspergillus* using MALDI FT-ICR MSI.[59] Also, like mycobacteria, the ability to characterize tissue distributions of antifungal drug levels may help guide clinical treatment of these infections.[60]

Perhaps the last, and arguably the most diverse, class of infectious pathogens is parasites, a broad class of organisms, ranging from intracellular Apicomplexa to larger multicellular organisms such as helminths, which have their own organ systems. Despite some similarities between humans and parasites, there are unique differences that could be leveraged to detect and identify these organisms in human tissue. Although there are a few examples of MSI applications to detect these organisms, this is an arguably underinvestigated field in MS, and MSI in particular, relative to its burden in humans. Perhaps the most prominent parasitic disease in terms of its public health burden in humans is malaria, which is caused by various *Plasmodium* species. *Plasmodium falciparum* is the deadliest species in humans, although there are numerous other *Plasmodium* species that infect both humans and other animals. Patterson and colleagues[61] used MALDI ionization MS to detect *Plasmodium yoelii*, which is used in murine models, to detect infection in liver, where these organisms spend part of their life cycle. Kadesch and colleagues[62] used atmospheric pressure scanning microprobe MALDI MS to detect *Toxoplasma gondii* and *Besnoitia besnoiti* in bovine monolayer cells. Although *B besnoiti* is an important pathogen in cattle, *T gondii* is an important human pathogen in immunocompromised patients as well as pregnant hosts because of the ability of *Toxoplasma* to cross the placenta and cause fetal disease. At present *T gondii* is detected in tissues either by histologic analysis with confirmation using PCR-based or IHC-based approaches. However, either of these approaches can take considerable time, and the ability to measure these organisms quickly and rapidly would be of value. Because of their focal nature in tissue, MSI could provide a metabolic or proteomic correlate to histology.

Although clinical MSI approaches have seen an emphasis on neoplastic disease, important applications for MSI in infectious diseases are reviewed here as well. The unique and xenobiotic nature of many of these biomolecules provides an ample opportunity for both the detection and identification of pathogens. Moreover, the ability to image these molecules within tissue using MSI provides the additional advantage of mapping the pathogen within the tissue and comparing it with histologic and immunohistochemical studies, which is generally not available with nucleic acid amplification approaches. The authors suspect this will be a rich area for clinical MSI applications in the coming years.

Analytical Parameters to Consider

The variety of ionization sources and mass analyzers and combinations therein provides a multitude of analytical setups to perform MSI. Each combination provides both advantages and disadvantages, and careful consideration of the clinical diagnostic question being asked should be taken before choosing any particular platform. As with any assay, general analytical parameters such as precision, accuracy, sensitivity, selectivity, stability, matrix effects, and interferences should be considered. Beyond these, there are several additional considerations that should also be considered with MALDI MSI (and MSI in general), including tradeoffs between sensitivity and specificity, throughput and resolution, as well as cost, ease of use, and other logistical and preanalytical factors, which are discussed later. Also, it is worth noting that, although MSI is a powerful analytical approach, regardless of the ionization and mass spectrometer used, simply using an imaging approach does not always provide additional clinical diagnostic benefits. A review and some perspective on the analytical parameters to consider in the context of the clinical scenario, available specimen, and diagnostic question being asked are provided here. For clinical applications, the optimal ionization method and mass spectrometer used may be guided by the clinical question to be answered and the analytical parameters needed to answer the question. Of course, additional factors, such as availability of equipment and expertise to run and perform such assays, are critical, although these are likely to change over time.

Preanalytical Considerations

As is true with many clinical diagnostic tests, preanalytical considerations are crucially important and often overlooked. First, most pathology specimens are either frozen or FFPE specimens. If frozen, there are a few specific considerations. One is that clinical specimens are generally embedded in optimal cutting temperature (OCT) media before being mounted and cut. Although this allows ideal sectioning in a cryostat, the OCT contains polymers that result in significant ion suppression in MALDI MSI and other MSI and MS methods. In the research setting, this can be avoided in a few ways: one is by not fully embedding the sample but by placing a small drop on which the specimen is mounted. In the clinical setting, this is very challenging, because many clinical samples are extremely small, and trying to mount and section these without embedding is impractical. Another option is using a different embedding medium that is compatible with MALDI. One study systematically tried several different embedding media and found that a supportive hydrogel was most effective and did not interfere with MALDI MSI.[63] Although using a different medium may be a long-term objective, the likelihood of changing what amounts to a nearly universal embedding/mounting medium is unlikely in the near future. Therefore, the most practical approach is removing the OCT before MSI analysis, which has been described using a technique that removes both OCT and salts, allowing better lipid analysis.[64] The other consideration is that fresh or frozen samples may still contain infectious agents, and processing poses a safety threat to people working with the specimens. Furthermore, enzymatic activity in the tissue can be reactivated during the thawing process, leading to activation of proteases, lipases, and other metabolic enzymes that will change the biochemical composition of the tissue. To avoid this, heating the tissue has been shown to both inactivate pathogens in the specimen as well as thermally inactivate the enzymes responsible for protein degradation.[65–67]

The other major specimen type is FFPE. Although the processes of formalin fixation, specimen processing, and paraffin embedding cause significant biochemical changes to the tissue, the benefit is that these specimens are biologically inactivated, and highly abundant, because they represent the largest number of specimens in most pathology departments and clinical biobanks. Despite its limitations, there has been considerable progress in processing and analysis using MALDI MSI, including enzymatic digestion by trypsin for bottom-up proteomic analysis or digestion by glycosidases for glycan analysis.[17,68–70] Regardless of whatever progress is made in working with fresh and frozen tissue, the potential to analyze the vast stores of pathology-banked FFPE tissues will continue to grow this area of development and MALDI MSI research.

Speed and Throughput Considerations

Clinical diagnostic workflows often require higher specimen throughput or shorter turnaround times than are demanded in most research settings. The considerable speed and multiplexing capacity has made MS very attractive in the clinical diagnostic space.[71] As such, assay speed is a critical feature for clinical implementation of MALDI MSI. However, when discussing speed, it is important to consider this in 2 contexts: (1) rapid workflows, and (2) high-throughput workflows.

Rapid workflows, like those needed in frozen section, where an urgent result is used for surgical guidance, the total time from sample collection to result is of utmost importance. Despite the promise of MALDI MSI, conventional methods can take an hour or more when considering matrix application and drying, image registration, and data acquisition. The authors have recently described a method to precoat and analyze a predetermined region containing the specimen with a high-frequency laser, allowing MALDI MSI, which conventionally takes anywhere from 30 minutes to 2 hours to prepare and analyze a slide, to take less than 5 minutes.[43]

In contrast, high-throughput workflows (eg, performing MALDI MSI for all surgical pathology specimens at a hospital) may not require each individual result to be performed rapidly but, because of the total number of samples, would still require a fast process to keep up with volume. To accomplish this, high-throughput MALDI MSI workflows can leverage performing preanalytical steps in parallel. For example, if deparaffinization, trypsinization, antigen retrieval, matrix application, or recrystallization are needed, these can be done for several samples at the same time. Therefore, by aligning and automating so-called latent preanalytical steps, high-throughput analysis may be possible.

Spatial Resolution

Perhaps the most powerful and distinguishing feature of MSI compared with other MS applications is the ability to preserve spatial relationship in tissue specimens. Spatial resolution is a parameter specific to imaging applications and can be roughly defined as the ability to distinguish 2 nearby points in an image and described by pixel size. The higher the spatial resolution, the smaller the pixel size.

There are several benefits of having high spatial resolution. First, spatial preservation prevents the dilution of lesional tissue with normal, inflammatory, or otherwise nonpathogenic tissue. One example in cancer is tumor staging, where detection of malignant cells within a lymph node can change the cancer stage. The challenge lies in that there may only be rare tumor cells within the lymph node. If the lymph node was processed in aggregate, it is possible that the signal from the cancer cells would not be detected. An example in a nonneoplastic disease is the detection of rare pathogens in tissue. For example, *M tuberculosis* can have an outsized impact in tissue with large granulomatous inflammation areas with only rare organisms present. Again, if the chemical signature of an infected tissue or even a smaller dissected region of inflammation were investigated, the microbial biochemical signature could be lost in normal or inflammatory tissue signal. High spatial resolution would allow much smaller pixel size and therefore significant advantages when analyzing such organisms. Dissection approaches, such as visually circling and scraping lesional tissue or using laser microdissection, can be used to enrich tumor content. However, MSI allows analysis directly on the tissue, precluding the need to dissect the tissue. This approach both reduces the time and labor required and provides much higher spatial resolution than can is possible with physical dissection.

Another benefit of high spatial resolution is in the analysis of heterogenous tissues. Many primary tumors, for example, can be very heterogenous, containing regions of lower and higher cellularity, and admixed with stromal and immune cells. Performing conventional MS analysis on homogenized or disaggregated tissues mixes the chemical signatures of these different cells and regions, resulting in both reduced sensitivity and specificity. Being able to preserve the spatial relationships between different areas of the tissues also allows merging these analyses with other modalities, such as histology, and immunohistochemistry, providing a more comprehensive and physiologic representation of the tissue as a system. However, one limitation, to higher spatial resolution is a relative decrease in sensitivity and increase in analytical time.

Spectral Resolution

In simplest terms, spectral resolution refers to the ability of the mass spectrometer to distinguish between 2 ions with close mass-to-charge ratio. The higher the mass spectral resolution, the more specific the mass identification. Incidentally, with the increased analytical specificity also comes increased analytical sensitivity because of a higher signal-to-noise ratio from fewer overlapping ions. There are several high-resolution MS platforms, including quadrupole TOF, Orbitrap and FT-ICR MS, the last of which can have a magnetic field as high as 21 T. There are several clinical applications in which high spectral resolution may be helpful. Most notably, most proteomic applications greatly benefit from the increased mass resolution to identify and quantify peptides. Also, this has been shown to be extremely helpful in drug analyses in tissue because of the high mass accuracy and improved signal-to-noise ratio for finding a particular drug or metabolite in tissue.

Much like spatial resolution, although it can be tempting to always want higher mass spectral resolution, there are tradeoffs as well. Perhaps the most challenging is the acquisition and maintenance of the equipment, which can be very expensive and require more technical expertise to run than lower-resolution instruments. Also, the mass resolution is only as good as its calibration and rigorous maintenance. For example, if a platform can distinguish down to 0.0001 Da, it likewise needs to be calibrated regularly to maintain this mass accuracy or it is not much more useful than a lower-resolution instrument. Note that most clinical MS that is currently performed in the clinical laboratory relies on the use of triple quadrupoles or TOF instruments, which function at lower or unit resolution. Despite this lower spectral resolution, LC-MS/MS has fundamentally transformed toxicology, therapeutic drug monitoring, inborn errors of metabolism, and other chemistry testing, and MALDI-TOF has transformed clinical microbiology microbe identification. Therefore, before opting for the highest resolving power, several issues, including the clinical need, the diagnostic question, as well as resources to both run and maintain such an instrument, must be considered.

SUMMARY AND FUTURE DIRECTIONS

As described in this article, there are numerous tissue-based clinical diagnostic applications for which MALDI MSI shows considerable promise. Not only has there been significant progress in cancer diagnostics but tissue-based infectious disease diagnostics represents another exciting area for expansion. Central to this progress will be consideration of the clinical workflows set up, and consequently which analytical parameters will be most important for the clinical diagnostic question being asked. Future applications include three-dimensional MALDI MSI, in which multiple slices of two-dimensional MALDI MSI data can be constructed to visualize another dimension of drug distribution.[72] Other areas of progress will be in drug distribution and pharmacokinetic studies, which are described in brief in this article.[47,73,74] This area is undoubtedly important in the evaluation and pharmaceutical development but may one day play a role in patient care as well. Progress in nonneoplastic and noninfectious processes such as amyloid diagnostics is also growing.[75,76] Just as MALDI-TOF MS changed microbial diagnostics in the microbiology laboratory, the authors anticipate MALDI MSI may have a similar impact in the coming years.

FUNDING

Support was provided by the National Institutes of Health/National Cancer Institute (NIH/NCI) Grant R01CA201469 and U54CA210180, the Breast Cancer Research Foundation, and the Ferenc Jolesz National Center for Image Guided Therapy at BWH (P41 EB015898).

CLINICS CARE POINTS

- MALDI MSI provides comprehensive molecular images of tissue.
- Recent developments allow rapid analysis.
- Further development is needed to expand the breadth of biomolecules detected.

REFERENCES

1. Buchberger AR, DeLaney K, Johnson J, et al. Mass spectrometry imaging: a review of emerging advancements and future insights. Anal Chem 2018;90(1): 240–65.
2. Ferguson CN, Fowler JWM, Waxer JF, et al. Mass spectrometry-based tissue imaging of small molecules. Adv Exp Med Biol 2019;1140:99–109.
3. Gode D, Volmer DA. Lipid imaging by mass spectrometry – a review. Analyst 2013. https://doi.org/10.1039/c2an36337b.
4. Gessel MM, Norris JL, Caprioli RM. MALDI imaging mass spectrometry: spatial molecular analysis to enable a new age of discovery. J Proteomics 2014;107: 71–82. https://doi.org/10.1016/j.jprot.2014.03.021.
5. Zhang J, Sans M, Garza KY, et al. Mass spectrometry technologies to advance care for cancer patients IN clinical and intraoperative use. Mass Spectrom Rev 2020. https://doi.org/10.1002/mas.21664.
6. Caprioli RM, Farmer TB, Gile J. Molecular imaging of biological samples: localization of peptides and proteins using MALDI-TOF MS. Anal Chem 1997;69(23): 4751–60.

7. Brender E. Frozen section biopsy. JAMA 2005. https://doi.org/10.1001/jama.294.24.3200.

8. Boskamp T, Lachmund D, Oetjen J, et al. A new classification method for MALDI imaging mass spectrometry data acquired on formalin-fixed paraffin-embedded tissue samples. Biochim Biophys Acta Proteins Proteom 2017;1865(7):916–26.

9. Angel PM, Bruner E, Bethard J, et al. Extracellular matrix alterations in low-grade lung adenocarcinoma compared with normal lung tissue by imaging mass spectrometry. J Mass Spectrom 2020;55(4):e4450.

10. Muranishi Y, Sato T, Ito S, et al. The ratios of monounsaturated to saturated phosphatidylcholines in lung adenocarcinoma microenvironment analyzed by liquid chromatography-mass spectrometry and imaging mass spectrometry. Sci Rep 2019;9(1):8916.

11. Dekker TJA, Balluff BD, Jones EA, et al. Multicenter matrix-assisted laser desorption/ionization mass spectrometry imaging (MALDI MSI) identifies proteomic differences in breast-cancer-associated stroma. J Proteome Res 2014;13(11):4730–8.

12. Torata N, Kubo M, Miura D, et al. Visualizing energy charge in breast carcinoma tissues by MALDI mass-spectrometry imaging profiles of low-molecular-weight metabolites. In: Anticancer research, vol. 38. International Institute of Anticancer Research; 2018. p. 4267–72. Available at: https://pubmed.ncbi.nlm.nih.gov/29970560/.

13. Angel PM, Schwamborn K, Comte-Walters S, et al. Extracellular matrix imaging of breast tissue pathologies by MALDI–imaging mass spectrometry. Proteomics Clin Appl 2019;13(1):e1700152.

14. Scott DA, Casadonte R, Cardinali B, et al. Increases in tumor N-glycan polylactosamines associated with advanced HER2-positive and triple-negative breast cancer tissues. Proteomics Clin Appl 2019;13(1):e1800014.

15. Balestrieri K, Kew K, McDaniel M, et al. Proteomic identification of tumor- and metastasis-associated galectin-1 in claudin-low breast cancer. Biochim Biophys Acta Gen Subj 2021;1865(2):129784.

16. Le Faouder J, Laouirem S, Chapelle M, et al. Imaging mass spectrometry provides fingerprints for distinguishing hepatocellular carcinoma from cirrhosis. J Proteome Res 2011;10(8):3755–65.

17. Powers TW, Neely BA, Shao Y, et al. MALDI imaging mass spectrometry profiling of N-glycans in formalin-fixed paraffin embedded clinical tissue blocks and tissue microarrays. PLoS One 2014. https://doi.org/10.1371/journal.pone.0106255.

18. Bien T, Perl M, Machmüller AC, et al. MALDI-2 mass spectrometry and immunohistochemistry imaging of Gb3Cer, Gb4Cer, and further glycosphingolipids in human colorectal cancer tissue. Anal Chem 2020;92(10):7096–105.

19. Sun C, Wang F, Wang X, et al. The choice of tissue fixative is a key determinant for mass spectrometry imaging based tumor metabolic reprogramming characterization. Anal Bioanal Chem 2020;412(13):3123–34.

20. Kunzke T, Balluff B, Feuchtinger A, et al. Native glycan fragments detected by MALDI-FT-ICR mass spectrometry imaging impact gastric cancer biology and patient outcome. Oncotarget 2017;8(40):68012–25.

21. Casadonte R, Kriegsmann M, Perren A, et al. Development of a class prediction model to discriminate pancreatic ductal adenocarcinoma from pancreatic neuroendocrine tumor by MALDI mass spectrometry imaging. Proteomics Clin Appl 2019;13(1):e1800046. https://doi.org/10.1002/prca.201800046.

22. Djidja MC, Claude E, Snel MF, et al. MALDI-ion mobility separation-mass spectrometry imaging of glucose-regulated protein 78 kDa (Grp78) in human

formalin-fixed, paraffin-embedded pancreatic adenocarcinoma tissue sections. J Proteome Res 2009;8(10):4876–84.

23. Randall EC, Zadra G, Chetta P, et al. Molecular characterization of prostate cancer with associated Gleason score using mass spectrometry imaging. Mol Cancer Res 2019;17(5):1155–65.

24. Schwamborn K, Krieg RC, Reska M, et al. Identifying prostate carcinoma by MALDI-imaging. Int J Mol Med 2007;20(2):155–9.

25. Cazares LH, Troyer D, Mendrinos S, et al. Imaging mass spectrometry of a specific fragment of mitogen-activated protein kinase/extracellular signal-regulated kinase kinase kinase 2 discriminates cancer from uninvolved prostate tissue. Clin Cancer Res 2009;15(17):5541–51.

26. Pallua JD, Schaefer G, Seifarth C, et al. MALDI-MS tissue imaging identification of biliverdin reductase B overexpression in prostate cancer. J Proteomics 2013;91: 500–14.

27. Goto T, Terada N, Inoue T, et al. The expression profile of phosphatidylinositol in high spatial resolution imaging mass spectrometry as a potential biomarker for prostate cancer. PLoS One 2014;9(2):e90242.

28. Wang X, Han J, Hardie DB, et al. Metabolomic profiling of prostate cancer by matrix assisted laser desorption/ionization-Fourier transform ion cyclotron resonance mass spectrometry imaging using Matrix Coating Assisted by an Electric Field (MCAEF). Biochim Biophys Acta Proteins Proteom 2017;1865(7):755–67.

29. Schwamborn K, Krieg RC, Uhlig S, et al. MALDI imaging as a specific diagnostic tool for routine cervical cytology specimens. Int J Mol Med 2011;27(3):417–21.

30. Pietkiewicz D, Horała A, Plewa S, et al. Maldi-msi—a step forward in overcoming the diagnostic challenges in ovarian tumors. Int J Environ Res Public Health 2020; 17(20):1–13.

31. Zhang H, Shi X, Vu NQ, et al. On-tissue derivatization with girard's Reagent P enhances N-glycan signals for formalin-fixed paraffin-embedded tissue sections in MALDI mass spectrometry imaging. Anal Chem 2020;92(19):13361–8.

32. Zhang C, Arentz G, Winderbaum L, et al. MALDI mass spectrometry imaging reveals decreased CK5 levels in vulvar squamous cell carcinomas compared to the precursor lesion differentiated vulvar intraepithelial neoplasia. Int J Mol Sci 2016; 17(7):1088.

33. Na CH, Hong JH, Kim WS, et al. Identification of protein markers specific for papillary renal cell carcinoma using imaging mass spectrometry. Mol Cells 2015;38(7):624–9.

34. Stella M, Chinello C, Cazzaniga A, et al. Histology-guided proteomic analysis to investigate the molecular profiles of clear cell Renal Cell Carcinoma grades. J Proteomics 2019;191:38–47.

35. Clark AR, Calligaris D, Regan MS, et al. Rapid discrimination of pediatric brain tumors by mass spectrometry imaging. J Neurooncol 2018;140(2):269–79.

36. Calligaris D, Feldman DR, Norton I, et al. MALDI mass spectrometry imaging analysis of pituitary adenomas for near-real-time tumor delineation. Proc Natl Acad Sci U S A 2015. https://doi.org/10.1073/pnas.1423101112.

37. Heijs B, Potthoff A, Soltwisch J, et al. MALDI-2 for the enhanced analysis of N-linked glycans by mass spectrometry imaging. Anal Chem 2020;92(20): 13904–11.

38. Agar NYR, Golby AJ, Ligon KL, et al. Development of stereotactic mass spectrometry for brain tumor surgery. Neurosurgery 2011. https://doi.org/10.1227/NEU.0b013e3181ff9cbb.

39. Louis DN, Perry A, Reifenberger G, et al. The 2016 World health Organization classification of tumors of the central nervous system: a summary. Acta Neuropathol 2016;131(6):803–20.

40. McDowell CT, Klamer Z, Hall J, et al. Imaging mass spectrometry and lectin analysis of N-linked glycans in carbohydrate antigen defined pancreatic cancer tissues. Mol Cell Proteomics 2020;20:100012.

41. Zhang J, Feider CL, Nagi C, et al. Detection of metastatic breast and thyroid cancer in lymph nodes by desorption electrospray ionization mass spectrometry imaging. J Am Soc Mass Spectrom 2017;28(6):1166–74.

42. Mittal P, Klingler-Hoffmann M, Arentz G, et al. Lymph node metastasis of primary endometrial cancers: associated proteins revealed by MALDI imaging. Proteomics 2016;16(11–12):1793–801.

43. Basu SS, Regan MS, Randall EC, et al. Rapid MALDI mass spectrometry imaging for surgical pathology. NPJ Precis Oncol 2019;3(1):17.

44. Santagata S, Eberlin LS, Norton I, et al. Intraoperative mass spectrometry mapping of an onco-metabolite to guide brain tumor surgery. Proc Natl Acad Sci U S A 2014;111(30):11121–6.

45. Keating MF, Zhang J, Feider CL, et al. Integrating the MasSpec pen to the da vinci surgical system for in vivo tissue analysis during a robotic assisted porcine surgery. Anal Chem 2020. https://doi.org/10.1021/acs.analchem.0c02037.

46. St John ER, Balog J, McKenzie JS, et al. Rapid evaporative ionisation mass spectrometry of electrosurgical vapours for the identification of breast pathology: towards an intelligent knife for breast cancer surgery. Breast Cancer Res 2017; 19(1):59.

47. Liu X, Ide JL, Norton I, et al. Molecular imaging of drug transit through the blood-brain barrier with MALDI mass spectrometry imaging. Sci Rep 2013. https://doi.org/10.1038/srep02859.

48. Jove M, Spencer J, Clench M, et al. Precision pharmacology: mass spectrometry imaging and pharmacokinetic drug resistance. Crit Rev Oncol Hematol 2019;141: 153–62.

49. Nishidate M, Hayashi M, Aikawa H, et al. Applications of MALDI mass spectrometry imaging for pharmacokinetic studies during drug development. Drug Metab Pharmacokinet 2019;34(4):209–16.

50. He Q, Sun C, Liu J, et al. MALDI-MSI analysis of cancer drugs: significance, advances, and applications. Trac Trends Anal Chem 2021;136:116183.

51. Bertzbach LD, Kaufer BB, Karger A. Applications of mass spectrometry imaging in virus research. In: Advances in virus research. Academic Press Inc; 2020. https://doi.org/10.1016/bs.aivir.2020.10.002.

52. Juříková T, Luptáková D, Kofroňová O, et al. Bringing SEM and MSI closer than ever before: visualizing Aspergillus and Pseudomonas infection in the rat lungs. J Fungi 2020;6(4):1–12.

53. Cox CR, Jensen KR, Saichek NR, et al. Strain-level bacterial identification by CeO2-catalyzed MALDI-TOF MS fatty acid analysis and comparison to commercial protein-based methods. Sci Rep 2015;5:10470.

54. Basu SS, McMinn MH, Giménez-Cassina Lopéz B, et al. Metal oxide laser ionization mass spectrometry imaging (MOLI MSI) using cerium(IV) oxide. Anal Chem 2019;91(10):6800–7.

55. Blanc L, Lenaerts A, Dartois V, et al. Visualization of mycobacterial biomarkers and tuberculosis drugs in infected tissue by MALDI-MS imaging. Anal Chem 2018;90(10):6275–82.

56. Prideaux B, Via LE, Zimmerman MD, et al. The association between sterilizing activity and drug distribution into tuberculosis lesions. Nat Med 2015;21(10): 1223–7.

57. Rychert J, Slechta ES, Barker AP, et al. Multicenter evaluation of the vitek MS v3.0 system for the identification of Filamentous fungi. J Clin Microbiol 2018; 56(2):1–11.

58. Lau AF, Drake SK, Calhoun LB, et al. Development of a clinically comprehensive database and a simple procedure for identification of molds from solid media by matrix-assisted laser desorption ionization-Time of flight mass spectrometry. J Clin Microbiol 2013;51(3):828–34.

59. Luptáková D, Pluháček T, Petřík M, et al. Non-invasive and invasive diagnoses of aspergillosis in a rat model by mass spectrometry. Sci Rep 2017;7(1):16523.

60. Zhao Y, Prideaux B, Baistrocchi S, et al. Beyond tissue concentrations: antifungal penetration at the site of infection. Med Mycol 2019;57(Supplement_2):S161–7.

61. Patterson NH, Tuck M, Lewis A, et al. Next generation histology-directed imaging mass spectrometry driven by autofluorescence microscopy. Anal Chem 2018; 90(21):12404–13.

62. Kadesch P, Hollubarsch T, Gerbig S, et al. Intracellular parasites Toxoplasma gondii and Besnoitia besnoiti, Unveiled in single host cells using AP-SMALDI MS imaging. J Am Soc Mass Spectrom 2020;31(9):1815–24.

63. Nelson KA, Daniels GJ, Fournie JW, et al. Optimization of whole-body zebrafish sectioning methods for mass spectrometry imaging. J Biomol Tech 2013;24(3): 119–27.

64. Truong JXM, Spotbeen X, White J, et al. Removal of optimal cutting temperature (O.C.T.) compound from embedded tissue for MALDI imaging of lipids. Anal Bioanal Chem 2021. https://doi.org/10.1007/s00216-020-03128-z.

65. Svensson M, Borén M, Sköld K, et al. Heat stabilization of the tissue proteome: a new technology for improved proteomics. J Proteome Res 2009;8(2):974–81.

66. Cazares LH, Van Tongeren SA, Costantino J, et al. Heat fixation inactivates viral and bacterial pathogens and is compatible with downstream MALDI mass spectrometry tissue imaging. BMC Microbiol 2015;15(1):101.

67. Ahnoff M, Cazares LH, Sköld K. Thermal inactivation of enzymes and pathogens in biosamples for MS analysis. Bioanalysis 2015;7(15):1885–99.

68. Diehl HC, Beine B, Elm J, et al. The challenge of on-tissue digestion for MALDI MSI- a comparison of different protocols to improve imaging experiments. Anal Bioanal Chem 2015. https://doi.org/10.1007/s00216-014-8345-z.

69. Holst S, Heijs B, De Haan N, et al. Linkage-specific in situ sialic acid derivatization for N-glycan mass spectrometry imaging of formalin-fixed paraffin-embedded tissues. Anal Chem 2016. https://doi.org/10.1021/acs.analchem. 6b00819.

70. Heijs B, Holst S, Briaire-De Bruijn IH, et al. Multimodal mass spectrometry imaging of N-glycans and proteins from the same tissue section. Anal Chem 2016. https://doi.org/10.1021/acs.analchem.6b01739.

71. Swiner DJ, Jackson S, Burris BJ, et al. Applications of mass spectrometry for clinical diagnostics: the influence of turnaround time. Anal Chem 2020;92(1): 183–202.

72. Abdelmoula WM, Regan MS, Lopez BGC, et al. Automatic 3D nonlinear registration of mass spectrometry imaging and magnetic resonance imaging data. Anal Chem 2019;91(9):6206–16.

73. Groseclose MR, Castellino S. A mimetic tissue model for the quantification of drug distributions by MALDI imaging mass spectrometry. Anal Chem 2013. https://doi.org/10.1021/ac400892z.
74. Castellino S, Groseclose MR. MALDI imaging mass spectrometry: bridging biology and chemistry in drug development. Bioanalysis 2011. https://doi.org/10.4155/bio.11.232.
75. Casadonte R, Kriegsmann M, Deininger S-O, et al. Imaging mass spectrometry analysis of renal amyloidosis biopsies reveals protein co-localization with amyloid deposits. Anal Bioanal Chem 2015. https://doi.org/10.1007/s00216-015-8689-z.
76. Winter M, Tholey A, Krüger S, et al. MALDI-mass spectrometry imaging identifies vitronectin as a common constituent of amyloid deposits. J Histochem Cytochem 2015. https://doi.org/10.1369/0022155415595264.

Moving?

Make sure your subscription moves with you!

To notify us of your new address, find your **Clinics Account Number** (located on your mailing label above your name), and contact customer service at:

Email: journalscustomerservice-usa@elsevier.com

800-654-2452 (subscribers in the U.S. & Canada)
314-447-8871 (subscribers outside of the U.S. & Canada)

Fax number: 314-447-8029

Elsevier Health Sciences Division
Subscription Customer Service
3251 Riverport Lane
Maryland Heights, MO 63043

*To ensure uninterrupted delivery of your subscription, please notify us at least 4 weeks in advance of move.

Printed and bound by CPI Group (UK) Ltd, Croydon, CR0 4YY

03/10/2024

01040400-0013